EMERGENCY GUIDE
FOR DENTAL AUXILIARIES

EMERGENCY GUIDE FOR DENTAL AUXILIARIES

Third Edition

Janet Bridger Chernega, MBA, MHA

DELMAR

THOMSON LEARNING ™

Australia Canada Mexico Singapore Spain United Kingdom United States

DELMAR
™
THOMSON LEARNING

Emergency Guide for Dental Auxiliaries 3e
by Janet Bridger Chernega

Health Care Publishing Director:
William Brottmiller

Executive Editor:
Cathy L. Esperti

Editorial Assistant:
Matthew Thouin

Executive Marketing Manager:
Dawn F. Gerrain

Channel Manager:
Jennifer McAvey

Production Editor:
Mary Colleen Liburdi

Cover Design:
William Finnerty

Library of Congress Cataloging-in-
Publication Data

ISBN 0-7668-1887-X

NOTICE TO THE READER

■ Contents

Chapter 9 Allergic Reactions

Chapter 10 Angina Pectoris and Myocardial Infarction

Chapter 11 Cardiopulmonary Resuscitation

Chapter 12 Cerebrovascular Accident

Chapter 13 Occupational Hazards and Emergencies

Chapter 14 Legal Problems of Emergency Care

■ Preface

Medical emergencies can and do occur within the dental office environment. A large percentage of these emergencies could be prevented or at least better treated if all the members of the dental team were more knowledgeable in the prevention and management of emergency situations.

The *Emergency Guide for Dental Auxiliaries* is designed to provide dental auxiliary students with the basic skills and knowledge necessary in order for each of them to function effectively as a member of the dental team. This text also will be an effective refresher tool for dental auxiliaries who are already working in dentistry.

The text includes objectives, review questions, and problem solving situations. This design should help the reader master new information as well as provide a format that will simplify review of previously learned materials.

The third edition of Emergency Guide for Dental Auxiliaries includes many new and updated topics such as latex allergies, gestational diabetes, Good Samaritan Laws, to name a few. In addition, new key words and expanded problem situations are included. The last chapter of the text provides information on the legal aspects of emergency case in the dental office. This chapter is designed as an overview. It is important that readers check the laws governing their own state for more detailed information.

Every effort has been made to ensure that the information in this text is accurate and up to date. However, due to the rapidly changing nature of both the dental and medical fields, the reader is encouraged to keep informed of changes announced by medical or dental authorities.

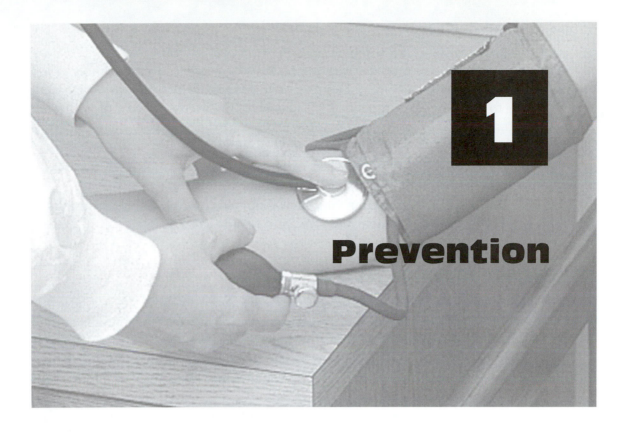

1

Prevention

KEY TERMS

Anticubital fossa
Blood pressure
Carotid artery
Diastolic pressure
Hypertension
Physician's Desk Reference
Pulse

Radial artery
Respiration rate
Sphygmomanometer
Stethoscope
Systolic pressure
Temperature

OBJECTIVES

Upon completion of this chapter the student will be able to:
- Name four vital signs
- Demonstrate the technique for recording each of these four vital signs
- Explain the normal range of each of the vital signs
- Explain the importance of having an accurate, updated health history for each dental patient
- Demonstrate the technique for completing and updating the health history
- Demonstrate the technique for utilizing the *Physician's Desk Reference (PDR)*

Most dental office emergencies can be prevented through the use of information found on thorough health histories. Dentists have found the easiest way to treat an emergency is to prevent it from occurring. This chapter discusses ways of gathering information that may help prevent an emergency.

VITAL SIGNS

The human body has certain vital signs that are important to measure: **blood pressure**, **pulse**, **respiratory rate**, and **temperature**.

BLOOD PRESSURE

Blood pressure is the pressure the blood places on the walls of the arteries. When there is too much pressure on the arteries, the patient suffers from **hypertension**, also known as high blood pressure. Hypertension can result in serious conditions such as stroke or cardiac arrest. By measuring blood pressure, the dentist may diagnose possible hypertension and prevent an emergency from occurring in the office.

Two readings are recorded when blood pressure is measured. The first reading is the **systolic pressure**, a measurement of the pressure on the arteries when the heart is beating, or working. The second reading is the **diastolic pressure**, which is a measurement of the pressure on the arteries when the heart relaxes between beats. If a patient reports a blood pressure reading of 120/80, the 120 represents the systolic pressure and the 80 the diastolic pressure.

To record blood pressure two items are needed: a **stethoscope** and a **sphygmomanometer**, which consists of a gauge and an inflatable bag inside a cloth armband (Figure 1-1). The sphygmomanometer is available in a range of sizes designed to fit children and adults. The cuff should always be selected according to the patient's size rather than the patient's age.

Technique

Blood pressure is measured by comparing the pressure in the artery with the air pressure in the armband using the following steps:

Step 1

- Expose the patient's arm. An accurate blood pressure cannot be taken over any type of clothing.

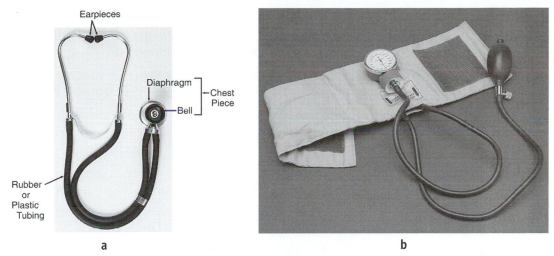

Figure 1-1 (a) Stethoscope and (b) sphygmomanometer

Step 2

- Select the cuff size. Be sure to select a size that fits snugly around the patient's arm without being tight enough to stop the flow of blood. A cuff that is too large or too small may produce an inaccurate reading.
- Place the cuff approximately an inch above the **anticubital fossa** (Figure 1-2).

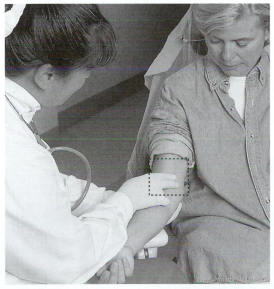

Figure 1-2 Location of the anticubital fossa

- Place the earpieces of the stethoscope into your ears. Make sure the earpieces are pointing toward the front of the head so that when they are placed in the ears, they follow the shape of the ear canal.

- Close the knob on the bulb by turning it clockwise. Be sure that the knob is not so tight as to prevent it from being easily turned with two fingers (Figure 1-3).

- Squeeze the bulb to pump air into the cuff until the pressure stops the flow of blood in the artery. This can be determined by palpating the **radial artery**. When no pulse is felt, the flow of blood has been stopped; this usually occurs around 180 mg Hg. At this point the pressure in the armband is higher than that in the artery, and the artery is squeezed shut.

- Place the stethoscope over the brachial artery (Figure 1-4).

- Turn the knob on the bulb counterclockwise slowly to release the pressure in the cuff. If the pressure is released too rapidly to hear the pulse sound, release all the pressure in the cuff and begin the procedure again.

- As soon as the cuff is loose enough to allow the blood to pass through the artery, you should hear a pulse. At this point the reading on the gauge is the systolic pressure.

- Continue to release the pressure in the cuff until a pulse is no longer heard. At this point the blood is flowing freely, and the reading on the gauge is of the diastolic pressure.

The technique described above is only one example of how to measure blood pressure. If you are in an office that utilizes a different technique, make sure you understand the steps involved and can perform the procedure accurately.

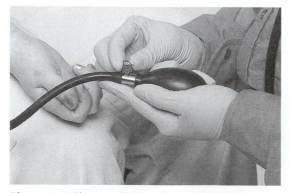

Figure 1-3 Close and open the knob on the blood pressure cuff

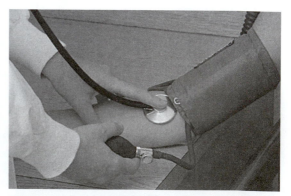

Figure 1-4 Placement of the stethoscope

Normal Readings

Physicians once considered 120/80 the normal range for blood pressure for adults, but most now believe that a lower reading is often acceptable. To determine what is normal for a particular patient, check the blood pressure over several visits to obtain a baseline reading. In addition, a consultation with the patient's physician may sometimes be indicated.

RECORDING THE PULSE

The pulse is also an important measurement to take on each dental patient. Measuring the pulse gives the dentist a very good picture of what is taking place with the patient's cardiac rhythm. As with any vital sign, it is important to have a baseline reading for comparison in the event of an emergency.

The pulse can be recorded at any major artery in the body. However, it is usually recorded at either the **carotid artery** or the radial artery. The radial artery, located in the wrist area, is usually the artery of choice for recording the pulse during a routine exam (Figure 1-5). It provides both easy access and an accurate reading. The carotid artery, located on either side of the neck, should be used to measure the pulse (Figure 1-6). When cardiac

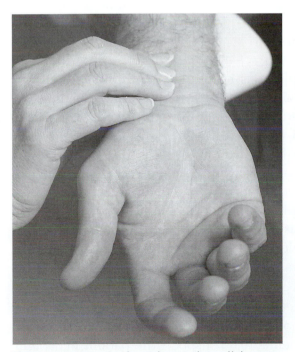

Figure 1-5 Measure the pulse at the radial artery

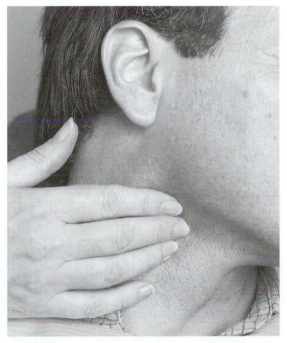

Figure 1-6 Measure the pulse at the carotid artery

output is very low because of an emergency condition, the pulse may be measured at the carotid artery when it is not palpable at the radial artery (the radial artery is peripheral, and blood flow usually ceases in that area first).

Technique

To record the pulse correctly, use the first and middle fingers. Place the two fingers firmly over the artery. Placing the fingers too lightly causes the beat of the pulse to be missed, but pressing too tightly cuts off the blood supply, eliminating the pulse altogether.

Once the artery has been located, count each beat of the pulse for a full minute. Observing the second hand of a watch is mandatory. Although the rate or speed of the pulse is important, attention must also be paid to the rhythm (regular or irregular) and to the quality (bounding or thready). Each of these readings is very important to the dentist in diagnosing the problem during an emergency. Although normal pulse readings vary among patients, for an adult the average range is 60 to 72 beats per minute.

RESPIRATION

The measurement of respirations involves counting the number of times the patient breathes in and out in one minute. An unusual **respiration rate** is a signal of possible emergency situations such as hyperventilation or certain cardiac problems.

To record the patient's respirations accurately, the patient should be unaware that someone is watching him breathe. Continue holding the patient's wrist as if the pulse is still being measure while actually watching and counting the rise and fall of the chest. As with the pulse, respirations should be measured for 60 seconds.

During cool weather when patients have on several layers of clothing, it is helpful to have the patient place one arm over the chest; the rise and fall of the arm then indicates the respirations. A normal range for respirations is 12 to 20 per minute, although this can be dramatically different among certain groups of people such as athletes.

TEMPERATURE

A patient's body temperature is not usually measured in the dental office on a routine basis. However, if the dental team suspects the patient may be ill, or if extensive surgery is to be performed, the dentist may request that the patient's body temperature be measured.

Use a thermometer to measure a patient's body temperature. An oral glass thermometer is most often used in a dental office. However, there are a variety of other types of thermometers, such as an electronic thermometer, a disposable paper thermometer, and a temperature-sensitive strip. The dental staff should select a thermometer that best meets their needs.

Technique

The oral route is recommended for routine temperature measurement in the dental office. The technique described below is for use with an oral glass thermometer. If other methods are utilized, follow the manufacturer's instructions.

1. Remove the thermometer from the storage container and rinse in cold water. Wipe dry with a tissue.
2. Check the reading on the thermometer. If it is not below 96 degrees F, shake the thermometer down until the mercury level is below that number.
3. Place the thermometer in the patient's mouth sublingually.
4. Instruct the patient to close the mouth and hold the thermometer in the mouth with the lips. Always caution the patient not to bite the glass thermometer.
5. Remove the thermometer from the patient's mouth and record the reading.
6. Clean the thermometer according to manufacturer's instructions.

Normal Readings

The normal reading for a child is 97-99, an adult is 97-99, and a geriatric patient (over 70 years old) is 96-99. See Table 1-1 for normal ranges of other vital signs.

HEALTH HISTORY

When a new patient enters the dental office, the staff and dentist seldom have any idea what types of medical problems he may have, and if an emergency arose, there would be no point of reference on which to base a probable diagnosis. The health history informs the staff of some possible problems to be prepared for as well as some drugs or treatments to avoid.

Table 1-1: Ranges for Normal Vital Signs

	BLOOD PRESSURE	PULSE	RESPIRATIONS	TEMP.
Infant	74-100/50-70	80-160	30-60	99.4-99.7
Preschool	82-110/50-78	80-120	22-34	98.6-99
School age	84-120/54-80	75-110	18-30	98-98.6
Adolescent	94-140/62-88	60-90	12-20	97-99
Adult	90-140/60-90	60-100	12-20	97-99
Geriatric (+70)	90-140/60-90	60-100	12-20	96-99

There is a great variety of patient health history forms, and most dental supply companies produce them. Many dentists design their own forms (Figure 1-7).

Health History Format

Regardless of what type of form the dental office uses, several sections are vital. First, the form should include a section for general information, including such items as name, age, address, telephone number, and person to contact in case of an emergency. The patient's physician should also be listed in case medical consultations are required.

The section on medical conditions is of utmost importance. Each condition should be listed by its common name so it will be easily understood by the patient.

Completing the Health History

The dental auxiliary or receptionist should always be available to help the patient complete the health history. Some patients prefer to complete the forms by themselves; others may not understand some of the terminology and may require assistance. As with any other information obtained in the dental office, the information on the health history is confidential.

MEDICAL HISTORY FORM

Please print.

Date: _____

Name_____ Home phone # _____

Address _____

City_____ State_____ Zip Code _____

Occupation_____ Work Phone _____

Date of Birth_____ Height_____ Weight_____ Sex: M   F

Closest Relative_____ Phone # _____

If you are completing this form for another person, what is your relationship to that person?

_____

How did you find out about our clinic?_____

For the following questions, circle yes or no, whichever applies. Your answers are for our records only and will be considered confidential. Please note that during your initial visit you will be asked some questions about your responses to this questionnaire and there may be additional questions concerning your health.

1. Are you in good health?   Yes   No

2. Has there been any change in your general health within the past year?   Yes   No

3. What was the date of your last physical examination?   _____

4. Are you now under the care of a physician?   Yes   No

    If yes, what is the condition being treated?   _____

5. Your physician's name and address   _____

6. Have you had any serious illness, injury or operation in the last five years?   Yes   No

    Have you been hospitalized in the last 5 years?   Yes   No

    If yes, what was the illness or problem?   _____

Figure 1-7 Example of a health history form (continues)

7. Please place a check beside any of the following diseases or conditions you have now or have had in the past.

__ Damaged heart valves	__ Fainting spells	__ Respiratory problems
__ Artificial heart valves	__ Seizures	__ Arthritis
__ Heart murmur	__ Persistent diarrhea	__ Stomach ulcer
__ Rheumatic heart disease	__ Recent weight loss/gain	__ Kidney disease
__ Heart disease	__ Diabetes	__ Tuberculosis
__ Heart attack	__ Type I	__ Persistent cough
__ Angina	__ Type II	__ Low blood pressure
__ High blood pressure	__ Gestational	__ Sexually transmitted
__ Arteriosclerosis	__ Liver disease	disease
__ Stroke	__ Blood transfusion	__ Epilepsy
__ Chest pain upon exertion	__ Tumor or growth	__ Mental health disorders
__ Short of breath after mild	__ Bulimia	__ Cancer
exertion	__ Anorexia	__ Immune disorders
__ Swollen ankles	__ Hepatitis A, B, or C	__ Herpes (Cold sores/fever
__ Congenital heart defect	__ Jaundice	blisters)
__ Cardiac pacemaker	__ AIDS	__ Night sweats
__ Sinus trouble	__ HIV infection	__ Blood disorders
__ Hay fever	__ Thyroid problems	__ Sickle cell or other
__ Asthma	__ Emphysema	anemias
__ Use of a bronchodilator	__ Bronchitis	

8. Please place a check if you are allergic or have every had a reaction to:

__ Local anesthetics	__ Sulfa drugs	__ Codeine or other
__ Penicillin or other	__ Aspirin	painkillers
antibiotics	__ Iodine	__ Barbiturates, sedatives
__ Latex or rubber items		

9. Are you allergic to anything not listed? If so, what _____

10. Have you had any serious problem associated with any previous dental treatment?   Yes   No

11. Do you wear the following:

    Contact lenses   Yes   No

    Removable dental appliances   Yes   No

12. Do you have any artificial implants, shunts, or artificial joint replacements?   Yes   No

    If yes, does your physician recommend antibiotics before dental treatment?   Yes   No

13. Do you have any disease, condition, or problem not listed above that you think I should know about?   Yes   No

_____

Figure 1-7 Example of a health history form (continued)

14. Are you now taking or have you evern taken diet drugs prescribed by your doctor (These would include, but are not limited to, Pondimin, Redux, Fen-phen, Phentermine, fenfluramine, dexfenfluramine)?   Yes   No

15. Are you taking Hormone Therapy?   Yes   No

16. Please provide the following information for any prescription and non-prescription medicine you are now taking:

Medicine's name	Beginning date	How often is the medicine taken?	Why do you take this medicine?

17. Circle if you are:

    Pregnant   Possibly pregnant, not sure   Nursing

18. Are you taking birth control pills or using other chemical means of birth control such as injections or implants (Norplant)?   Yes   No

19. What is your chief dental need or problem?   _____

I certify that I have read and understand all of the questions above. I acknowledge that my questions, if any, about the questions set forth above have been answered to my satisfaction. I will not hold the dentist, or any other member of his/her staff, responsible for any errors or omissions that I may have made in the completion of this form.

Patient's Signature _____**Date**_____

Parent/Guardian's Signature _____**Date**_____

Figure 1-7 Example of a health history form (continued)

Updating the Health History

Each time the patient returns to the office for a routine visit, the health history should be updated. A person's medication or medical condition can change very rapidly, and it is extremely important to keep this information current.

Using the Physician's Desk Reference

After reviewing the patient's medical history, the auxiliary should research in a drug reference source any medications the patient is currently taking. This is extremely valuable to the entire dental team in understanding existing medical conditions, preventing improper mixtures of medications, and determining if there are restrictions as to the type of treatment that may be provided to the patient.

Several sources may be utilized to obtain this information. The dentist and staff should decide which source best meets the needs of their office.

One good drug reference source is the *Physician's Desk Reference (PDR)*. The *PDR* is compiled annually and contains information provided by the drug manufacturers about a large variety of medications. Several sections are color coded and may be of value to the auxiliary. Complete instructions on how to use each section are provided at the beginning of the section.

The produce identification section provides pictures of a wide variety of medications. Often, a patient comes to the office with a pill box containing a variety of medications, but the patient does not know the names of the medications and often does not know the condition for which the medications have been prescribed. This section allows the auxiliary to visually identify the medication. Even though it is ultimately the dentist's responsibility to make all decisions regarding the patient's medications, it is important for the auxiliary to know as much as possible about the patient to assist in providing proper treatment.

The auxiliary should become familiar with the contents of the drug reference source selected, and should utilize it regularly. It is also extremely important to have an up-to-date resource, because medications change at such a rapid pace.

SUMMARY

Vital signs such as blood pressure, pulse, respiration, and temperature are an excellent means of determining the patient's current medical status. In addition, the health history informs the dentist of past and present medical conditions. When they have all this information available, the doctor and staff have taken the first step toward preventing serious dental office emergencies.

REFERENCES

Cantrell, James R. (January 1982). Evaluation of the patient during a medical emergency. *Dental Clinics of North America, 26.*

Craven, Ruth F., and Constance J. Hirnle. (1992). *Fundamentals of nursing: Human health and function.* Lippincott.

Dental assistant's career advancement program. (1982). Procom.

Malamed, Stanley F. (1982). *Handbook of medical emergencies in the dental office* (2nd ed.). St. Louis: Mosby.

McCarthy, Frank M. (1982). *Medical emergencies in dentistry: An abridged edition of emergencies in dental practice* (3rd ed.). Philadelphia: Saunders.

Waisbern, Burton A. (1973). *Emergency care manual: A systemic approach.* Flushing, NY: Medical Examination Publishing Co.

REVIEW QUESTIONS

MULTIPLE CHOICE

1. Which of the following is/are considered a vital sign?
   a. temperature
   b. vision
   c. pulse
   d. a and c, only

2. Which of these are needed to record blood pressure?
   a. sphygmomanometer
   b. thermometer
   c. stopwatch
   d. all the above

3. Which artery is used to measure blood pressure?
   a. femoral
   b. carotid
   c. radial
   d. brachial ✓

4. What artery is *usually* used to record the pulse during an emergency?
   a. radial
   b. carotid ✓
   c. femoral
   d. brachial

5. Respirations should be measure for _____ seconds.
   a. 30
   b. 15
   c. 10
   d. none of the above ✓

TRUE OR FALSE

F 1. The health history should only be taken on emergency patients.
T 2. The health history should be updated each time the patient comes to the office.
F 3. A normal range for respirations is 60 to 72.
F 4. The thumb and first finger should be used to record the pulse because they do not have a pulse of their own.
F 5. Blood pressure may be recorded through any type of clothing.
F 6. The *Physician's Desk Reference* should be replaced every year.

2

Office Preparation

KEY TERMS

Ampule
Demand-valve resuscitator
Emergency kit
Flowmeter

Nasal canula
Oxygen tank
Regulator

OBJECTIVES

Upon completion of this chapter the student will be able to:

- Explain the role of the dental auxiliary during an office emergency
- Explain the importance of an office emergency routine
- Describe the functions of the auxiliary in relation to the emergency kit
- Identify the attachments used with an oxygen tank
- Explain the importance of the demand-valve resuscitator
- Demonstrate the operation of the oxygen tank

Regardless of how much care is taken, not all dental office emergencies can be prevented. Therefore, should an emergency occur, the staff must be prepared. Being prepared includes having a well-planned emergency routine, having available all necessary equipment, and posting emergency numbers by all phones.

OFFICE EMERGENCY ROUTINE

To prevent a minor office emergency from becoming serious or perhaps even fatal, it is important to have a thorough office emergency routine—a definitive plan that indicates the functions and responsibilities of each member of the dental team.

Role of the Dental Auxiliary

Every dental office varies in the responsibilities designated for each person, however, here are six possible responsibilities that may be delegated to the dental auxiliary:

1. *Notify the dentist of the emergency.* The dentist is responsible for everything in his or her office and must be notified immediately.
2. *Administer basic life support if necessary.* Basic life support consists of maintaining an open airway, providing artificial respiration, and providing external cardiac compressions. All auxiliaries should be able to provide basic life support if needed.
3. *Retrieve the **emergency kit**.* Once an emergency situation is identified, the emergency kit should be brought to the area immediately so that all the available equipment is ready to be used.
4. *Retrieve the oxygen tank.* Oxygen is useful in most emergency situations. Have it available even if the cause or type of emergency has yet to be diagnosed.
5. *Retrieve hard backboard.* CPR cannot be performed on a soft dental chair, and many offices therefore have available a piece of board that fits underneath the patient in the back of the dental chair. This board should be brought to the chair in case CPR becomes necessary. If a backboard is not available, the patient must be placed on the floor of the operatory.
6. *Assist the dentist by preparing emergency drugs.* Although it is not legal for auxiliaries to administer drugs, it is legal in some states for them to prepare the drugs for the dentist to administer. This is helpful in situations where several drugs must be given in succession.

Role of the Receptionist

The receptionist, although not usually in direct contact with the patient, has several responsibilities during an emergency.

1. The receptionist should have all emergency numbers updated and within easy reach. It is an excellent idea always to keep these numbers posted close to the telephone.
2. Notify the emergency unit. When contacting the emergency rescue unit, the receptionist should report the nature of the emergency and give explicit directions to the office.
3. Go outside to direct emergency personnel into the office—this saves valuable time.

   Checklist for calling in an emergency:
   - State that your need for the rescue unit is an emergency.
   - Explain the nature of the emergency.
   - Give the name of the injured person.
   - Give the age of the victim.
   - Specify the exact location.
   - Give your name
   - Give your telephone number
   - Stay on the line until the operator instructs you to hang up.

4. Keep waiting room patients calm. If the emergency is serious, the patients in the waiting room should be rescheduled. Depending on the circumstances, this can be handled while they are in the office, or the receptionist may call the patients later. The waiting patients should be informed that there is an emergency situation but should not be given information concerning the nature of the emergency or the patient's name.

Anyone in the office may be assigned these tasks. The important thing is that each person understands exactly what his or her responsibilities involve.

Practice Routine

Once everyone understands his or her responsibilities, the emergency routine must be practiced on a regular basis. An emergency should be simulated, with each person performing his or her assigned functions. A well-prepared staff handles an emergency much more efficiently than one that has not had practice drills.

EMERGENCY KIT

Types

There are several types of emergency kits. One type that is gaining popularity is the homemade emergency kit. The homemade kit is usually assembled by the dentist with the help of physicians, pharmacists, and other medical personnel. This type of kit may be stored in a large fishing tackle box, on a set of instrument trays, or in a cart specifically designed for the purpose by several dental companies. The advantages of the homemade kit are:

1. The dentist knows exactly what is in the kit and is thus more likely to be able to use each piece of equipment and each drug proficiently.
2. The kit is designed by the dentist to meet his or her particular needs.

The second type of emergency kit is the manufactured kit, made in a variety of styles and available from every major dental supply company. The advantages of the manufactured kit are:

1. It comes in a carrying case that has compartments specially designed for each item.
2. It is designed specifically for dental office emergencies.
3. The kit is color coded to match the equipment or drugs with a particular type of emergency.
4. Some kits are available with pre-filled syringes which provide rapid emergency response.
5. Kits are available with automatic replacement of outdated medications.
6. Kits may come with emergency training videos.

The main disadvantage is that an elaborate manufactured kit sometimes contains some equipment or drugs with which the dentist is not completely familiar.

The key to selecting the correct type of emergency kit for any dental office is to make sure it meets the dentist's needs. For example, if the office is located a great distance from any medical facility, the dentist would require a fairly elaborate emergency kit, whereas the dentist located across the street from a hospital would require a minimal amount of emergency equipment.

See table for sample emergency kit contents.

The Dental Auxiliary and the Emergency Kit

Auxiliaries may feel they do not need to be concerned about the emergency kit, since in most areas it is illegal for the auxiliary to use the majority of the

Table 2-1: Sample Emergency Kit Contents

Ampule Epinephrine
Ampule Aminophylline
Ammonia inhalants
Ampule Atropine
Bottle of Nitrostat
Mix-o-vial Solu-Cortef
Ampule Talwin
Ampule Tigan
Ampule Diazepam
Ampule Wyamine
Ampule Benadryl
12 cc disposable syringe
3 cc disposable syringe
Tourniquet
12 gauge tracheotomy needle
Plastic airway

items in the kit. Actually, the auxiliary should be thoroughly familiar with each piece of equipment and each drug in the emergency kit. Auxiliaries can be a tremendous help during an emergency by preparing the correct drug or equipment promptly.

In addition, it should be the auxiliary's responsibility to inspect the kit on a routine basis to check for broken equipment and expired or depleted drugs. Drugs should always be kept updated (Figure 2-1). Administering an outdated drug used during an emergency could prove fatal. If the dentist wishes, arrangements can be made with certain pharmaceutical companies to replace the drugs automatically before they reach their expiration date. If such an arrangement is made, the dates should still be double-checked by the auxiliary to prevent any errors.

The auxiliary should become very familiar with the dental office's emergency kit. If the kit was ordered from a manufacturer, instructions should be included. However, if the kit was assembled by the dentist, special instructions may be required from other sources.

Most manufactured kits contain drugs in single-dose **ampules** (Figure 2-1). These ampules are designed to make it easy for the dental team to prepare an injection during an emergency situation. To open the ampule, hold the ampule with both hands and break it open at the color-coded line. Be careful to hold the ampule upright when breaking it open to prevent spillage. Once the ampule is open, the top portion can be discarded, and the auxiliary can load the syringe from the remaining portion of the ampule.

Location

The emergency kit should always remain in one location that is known by everyone in the office. The kit should also be easily accessible to everyone in the office.

OXYGEN TANK

Oxygen is one item that can easily be administered by anyone trained in its use and is extremely useful in most emergency situations except hyperventilation.

Tank

The oxygen comes in a cylinder. All **oxygen tanks** are green, which distinguishes oxygen from other gas. The cylinders range in size from very large to so small it can be carried in the hand. Letters of the alphabet have been chosen to specify certain sizes of oxygen tanks; the size best for the dental office is the E cylinder. This contains about 650 liters of oxygen and provides 100 percent oxygen for 30 minutes of constant use.

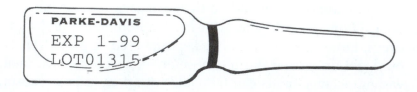

Figure 2-1 Expiration date on a drug ampule

Attachments

When the oxygen tank comes from the manufacturer, it consists only of the cylinder. A device known as a **regulator** must be attached to this tank so oxygen may be administered to the patient. The regulator is placed onto the tank to allow the pressure to be released at a reduced rate (Figure 2-2). Once the regulator is in place, the flow of oxygen can be adjusted by using a **flowmeter** that controls the amount of oxygen given to the patient. The two main types used are the bourbon gauge flowmeter and the pressure-compensated flowmeter. The bourbon gauge consists of a round dial that indicates the flow of oxygen in liters per minute. Although it is a pressure gauge and may therefore sometimes give inadequate readings when low amounts of oxygen are administered, it is found on a majority of tanks used in dental offices and can be very functional.

The pressure-compensated flowmeter consists of a vertical glass tube with a ball float that rises and falls with the flow of oxygen going through the tube. This gauge indicates the actual flow at all times. Because it depends on the force of gravity, it must always be operated in an upright position.

These valves and gauges are necessary to release oxygen from the tank, but extra attachments are required to administer oxygen to the patient.

The vast number of such attachments available range from **nasal canulas** to full oxygen tents. However, a basic mask should be sufficient for administering oxygen during an emergency situation in a dental office. The mask must meet specific criteria to be effective. First, it must fit the face of the patient so as to provide a tight seal (Figure 2-3). Oxygen masks come in a variety of sizes ranging from pedo to adult and should be available in every

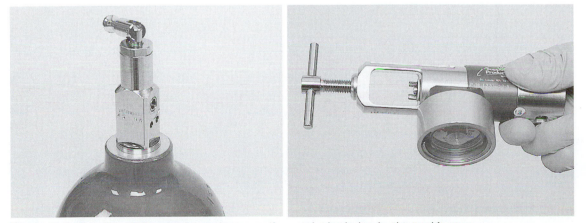

Figure 2-2 The pins of the regulator must exactly match the holes in the tank's stem.

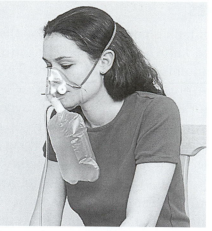

Figure 2-3 Properly fitting clear face mask

dental office. Second, the mask should be made of a clear substance. It is imperative that the patient be monitored during oxygen administration to make sure she does not vomit into the mask and then aspirate the vomitus into her lungs. Furthermore, with a clear mask the person administering the oxygen can tell when the patient has begun to breathe on her own because the mask will fog.

Another extremely important attachment for the office oxygen tank is the **demand-valve resuscitator**. The regular office oxygen tank is of no use on a patient who is not breathing, because there is no way to force the oxygen into the lungs. This is the function of the demand-valve resuscitator. The demand valve consists of a pushbutton, located on the face mask, that controls the flow of oxygen. When the button is pressed, oxygen goes through the mask with enough force to inflate the lungs. It continues to force oxygen into the lungs until it reaches a preset pressure, at which point it stops. The demand valve is very beneficial during CPR because it provides 100 percent oxygen rather than the oxygen-carbon dioxide mix a human could provide. Furthermore, if the patient starts breathing, it automatically provides oxygen when the person inhales and stops when she exhales.

Other less-expensive items such as the ambubag may be used in place of the demand valve. The most important consideration is to have some mechanism available to force oxygen into the lungs of the nonbreathing victim.

Operating the Tank

When operating an oxygen tank, follow these steps:

1. When opening a new tank, use the attached wrench and crack the seal to release a little oxygen to clear dust and debris from the valves.
2. Attach the regulator and flowmeter, which are designed with specific grooves and holes so they can only go on one way.
3. Open the regulator valve all the way and then turn it back one turn. This prevents someone from thinking it is closed and damaging the equipment by turning it the wrong way.
4. Adjust the flowmeter to the point at which it is releasing 4 to 6 liters of oxygen.
5. Check the face mask hose to make sure there are no twists or knots.
6. Place the mask over the patient's face. Make sure the mask fits the patient with a good seal.
7. When oxygen therapy is completed, remove the face mask, turn the flowmeter to zero, and close the tank valve. Be sure to clean or to dispose of it, depending on the manufacturer's instructions.

Precautions

Although oxygen is a relatively safe gas to administer, a few precautions should be followed in the dental office:

1. Do not use oxygen near an open flame. Oxygen is very flammable, and although it will not burn itself, it will make a small flame burn out of control.
2. Grease or oil of any kind will make the oxygen explode. Make sure you do not have oil on your hands when you operate the tank and that the tank is not stored around dirty, oily rags.

SUMMARY

Emergencies do occur in even the best-prepared dental office. However, a staff that knows what its responsibilities are, has all the equipment available, and knows how to use it can often prevent minor emergencies from becoming major emergencies.

REFERENCES

Grant, Harvey, and Robert Murray. *Emergency Care*. 2nd ed. Bowie, Md.: Robert J. Brady Co., 1978.

Malamed, Stanley P. *Handbook of Medical Emergencies in the Dental Office*. 2nd ed. St. Louis: Mosby, 1982.

Morrow, G.T. "Designing of a Drug Kit." *Dental Clinics of North America* 28 (January 1982).

REVIEW QUESTIONS

MULTIPLE CHOICE

1. During an office emergency, which of the following is not a function of the dental auxiliary?
   a. notify the doctor
   b. administer basic life support
   c. administer necessary drugs
   d. retrieve the emergency kit

2. All oxygen tanks are
   a. green
   b. blue
   c. red
   d. yellow

3. The amount of oxygen the patient receives is controlled by the
   a. regulator
   b. demand valve
   c. cylinder
   d. flowmeter

4. Grease or oil should not be used around oxygen because it will
   a. contaminate the oxygen
   b. cause an explosion
   c. block the valves
   d. none of the above

5. Which of the following is/are true concerning the face mask on the oxygen tank?
   a. should be clear
   b. should form a tight seal
   c. should be made of metal
   d. a and b

TRUE OR FALSE

T 1. The emergency kit should be easily accessible to everyone in the office.
T 2. Dental auxiliaries may administer oxygen if they are trained in its use.
F 3. The expiration date on drugs found in the emergency kit can be checked only by the dentist.
T 4. An E-cylinder oxygen tank should be used in the dental office.
T 5. When you are administering oxygen, the flowmeter should be set on 4-6 liters.

■ CASE STUDY

While receiving dental treatment, Mr. Jones, a 45-year-old with a history of heart problems, loses consciousness and goes into cardiac arrest. The doctor sends the auxiliary to the front to call for help while he goes to hook up the new oxygen cylinder that had arrived that morning. At the front desk, the assistant asks the receptionist to find the number for the rescue squad. When the doctor and assistant return to the operatory, they begin two-person CPR with the patient in the dental chair.

QUESTION

1. List everything that was done incorrectly.
2. List the correct steps.

3

Vasodepressor Syncope

KEY TERMS

Nonpsychogenic
Presyncope
Psychogenic
Supine position

Syncope
Trendelenburg position
Vasodepressor syncope

OBJECTIVES

Upon completion of this chapter the student will be able to:

- Define vasodepressor syncope
- Describe the causes of vasodepressor syncope
- Describe the physiology of vasodepressor syncope
- Explain ways to prevent vasodepressor syncope
- List the signs and symptoms of vasodepressor syncope
- Demonstrate the treatment for vasodepressor syncope

The most common life-threatening emergency that may be experienced in the dental office is *vasodepressor syncope* (better known as the common faint), a loss of consciousness caused by a decrease in the blood flow to the brain. Although vasodepressor syncope is a fairly common occurrence, if not promptly corrected it can lead to death. As a result, it has been suggested that all episodes of unconsciousness should be treated as cardiac arrest until otherwise diagnosed.

CAUSES

Vasodepressor syncope is most often caused by some form of stress—physical, emotional, or both. For descriptive purposes, these causes have been categorized as either **psychogenic** or **nonpsychogenic**. Psychogenic factors are psychological causes; nonpsychogenic factors are physical causes. Psychogenic factors include fear, pain, emotional upset, and anxiety that can be specifically related to the dental office in the following ways:

1. Most dental patients have some degree of fear about dental treatment. When this fear becomes overwhelming and unmanageable, it can become a psychogenic cause of vasodepressor syncope.
2. All the modern advances have come close to making routine dentistry a painless experience. Even so, in some situations (inadequate anesthesia, for example) pain may be experienced. This type of sudden pain may cause vasodepressor syncope.
3. Unfortunately, there are times the dentist has to inform the patient of a poor prognosis. Bad news can sometimes trigger in some patients an emotional upset severe enough to cause vasodepressor syncope.

Psychogenic factors are the most common causes of vasodepressor syncope in the dental office.

Nonpsychogenic factors include hunger, poor health, and remaining in an upright position for a long period. Although nonpsychogenic factors can certainly cause syncope, they are experienced in the dental office much less often than psychogenic factors.

PHYSICAL CHANGES RESULTING IN VASODEPRESSOR SYNCOPE

Once certain psychogenic or nonpsychogenic factors are present, changes within the body may result in vasodepressor syncope. First, the body experiences some type of stress (pain, fear, or the like). As a result, certain products in the body trigger a reaction that causes a dilation of the vascular bed, resulting in large amount of blood being pumped—mainly to the muscles of the arms and legs (the "fight or flight" syndrome). Since the patient remains stationary in the dental chair, this extra blood is not recirculated adequately and tends to pool in the arms and legs, resulting in a deficiency of blood to the heart and thus a lack of oxygenated blood going to the brain. As a result of the brain's deprivation of adequate oxygen, unconsciousness occurs.

SIGNS AND SYMPTOMS

Vasodepressor syncope usually occurs with the patient in an upright position, such as sitting upright in the dental chair. Vasodepressor syncope is a relatively slow-occurring problem, usually passing through different stages, each of which exhibits distinctive signs and symptoms. **Presyncope**, the first stage, precedes actual loss of consciousness (see Emergency Basics). During this stage the patient is pale and covered in cold sweat, and may complain of being hot, dizzy, or nauseated. Vital signs at this time show a slight decrease in blood pressure and a very rapid increase in pulse. The decrease in blood pressure is due to the dilation of the vessels, and the increase in pulse rate is due to the heart working so hard to send the extra blood to the body periphery. The heart can only work this hard for a short period. Once it tires, it no longer circulates a sufficient amount of blood. Therefore the blood pressure and pulse rate drop rapidly immediately before the patient advances to the **syncope** stage.

Syncope, the next stage, consists of the actual loss of consciousness (Emergency Basics). During this stage, the patient exhibits a deathlike appearance, the breathing may be shallow and gasping, slight convulsive movements may be present, and pupils are dilated. Vital signs monitored at this time show a very low blood pressure and a slow and thready pulse.

TREATMENT

Remain calm. During syncope, as in all emergencies, the dental team must remain calm and in control. The patient who revives and sees a very nervous and upset support group could very easily have a relapse. As soon as you suspect that patient is experiencing vasodepressor syncope, stop all dental treatment. The old idea of having the patient place the head between the knees is no longer accepted as a means of treatment. Placing the head between the knees makes it more difficult to breathe; in this position the patient's brain does not receive adequate oxygen—which caused the episode in the first place. Instead, place the patient in the **Trendelenburg position** (Figure 3-1). The Trendelenburg position is a **supine position** with the feet slightly elevated. Since most dental patients are already in the supine position, this

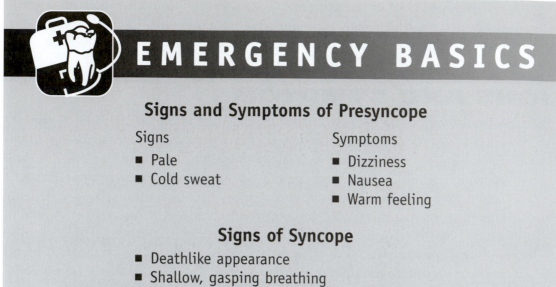

EMERGENCY BASICS

Signs and Symptoms of Presyncope

Signs
- Pale
- Cold sweat

Symptoms
- Dizziness
- Nausea
- Warm feeling

Signs of Syncope
- Deathlike appearance
- Shallow, gasping breathing
- Dilated pupils
- Convulsive movements (possible)

is easily achieved by slightly lowering the back of the chair. Placing the patient in this reclining position helps alleviate syncope because gravity is no longer a factor in getting blood to the brain. If the patient loses consciousness in the waiting room or hallway, place the patient supine on the floor and elevate the legs slightly. This may be accomplished by placing an object such

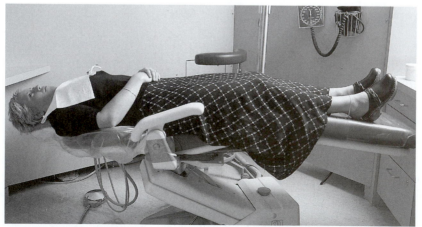

Figure 3-1 Trendelenburg position

as a chair, coat, pillow, or the like under the feet or simply by holding the legs in an elevated position.

Properly positioning the patient is the most important step in treating syncope and should be followed in every case except when dealing with a pregnant patient. If the pregnant patient is placed in the Trendelenburg position, the weight of the fetus pressing against the diaphragm may inhibit breathing. So the pregnant patient should be placed on her side before elevating the feet. Once properly positioned, the patient should recovery rapidly. If recovery does not occur right away, the next step is to make sure the patient has an open airway.

When a person loses consciousness, the muscles of the tongue relax and the tongue may fall to the back of the throat, blocking the airway. When the airway is blocked, no oxygen goes to the brain, and the patient could die. To open the airway, utilize the head tilt/chin lift techniques described in the section on cardiopulmonary resuscitation (Chapter 11).

Once the airway is opened, the patient should begin to breathe on his own. If he does not, other causes of unconsciousness must be considered, and more extensive treatment may be required.

With the patient properly positioned and the airway open, an ammonia capsule may be cracked and passed quickly back and forth under the patient's nose to help stimulate breathing. Pure oxygen via full face mask may also be administered to aid in breathing. The vital signs should begin to return to their baseline readings. Furthermore, anything that can be done to help make the patient more comfortable should be done. This includes loosening tight clothing, placing a cold towel on the forehead, or providing some type of covering if the patient complains of being cold once he begins to recover.

On first recovering, the patient may be slightly confused and upset. The situation should be explained in a very calm, reassuring manner. Some patients may be embarrassed by the episode; if so, extra efforts should be made to put the patient at ease.

A patient who has fainted may faint again very soon after recovery. Therefore it is very important to remove any predisposing stimuli such as needles, blood, and the like from the patient's sight. Whether dental treatment will continue will have to be decided by the doctor and the patient. Whatever the decision, the patient needs some time to recover and should be kept calm and quiet. Also, the patient should not be left unattended. A patient who has lost consciousness in the dental chair should not be moved until fully recovered. Of course, if the episode occurred in the waiting room or hallway, it would be best, once consciousness has returned, to move the patient to a more appropriate area in which to recover.

Once the patient has recovered completely, all the information concerning the episode should be documented in the patient's chart, including the signs and symptoms exhibited and the treatment provided. An example of treatment is shown in the following Emergency Basics.

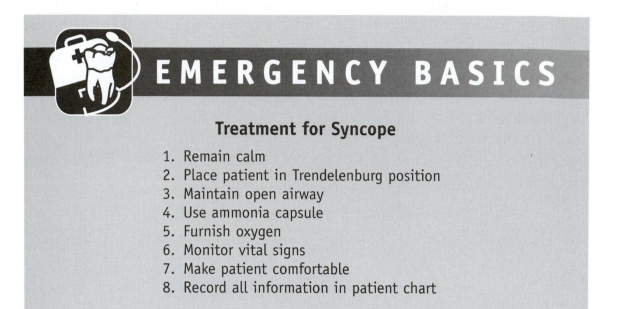

EMERGENCY BASICS

Treatment for Syncope

1. Remain calm
2. Place patient in Trendelenburg position
3. Maintain open airway
4. Use ammonia capsule
5. Furnish oxygen
6. Monitor vital signs
7. Make patient comfortable
8. Record all information in patient chart

PREVENTION

If the signs and symptoms of presyncope are noted early enough, in most instances you can prevent the patient from ever advancing to the full syncope stage. When such signs and symptoms as cold sweat, nausea, or dizziness are present, stop dental treatment and place the patient in the Trendelenburg position. Also try to remove or alleviate whatever caused the patient distress in the first place. In most cases the patient will recover completely.

Furthermore, it is possible to prevent any signs and symptoms of any phase of vasodepressor syncope.

Since fear or anxiety is the most common cause of vasodepressor syncope in the dental office, the easiest way to prevent syncope is to alleviate the fear. This can be achieved by doing everything possible to make the patient comfortable and may include talking with the patient, providing a bright, cheery atmosphere, or alleviating unpleasant sounds and smells associated with the dental office. In some cases it might be helpful to premedicate the patient to alleviate extreme anxieties.

Syncope may also be prevented by maintaining a thorough, updated health history. The patient who has a history of syncope is very likely to experience it during the dental visit. If the staff can find out what causes the person to faint, extra precautions can be taken to prevent the patient from experiencing these conditions.

SUMMARY

By being familiar with the patient's history and taking extra effort to reduce stress in the dental office, the auxiliary can prevent most cases of vasodepressor syncope from ever occurring. However, in the event syncope does occur, the well-trained auxiliary can correct a potentially life-threatening emergency by following the basic treatment of Trendelenburg position, maintaining an open airway, and administering oxygen and ammonia.

REFERENCES

Harrison, John B. "Faints and Spells." *Dental Clinics of North America 17* (July 1973).

Hendler, Barry R., and Louis F. Rose. "Common Medical Emergencies: A Dilemma in Dental Education." *Journal of the American Dental Association 91* (September 1975).

Malamed, Stanley F. *Handbook of Medical Emergencies in the Dental Office.* 2nd ed., St. Louis: Mosby, 1982.

McCarthy, Frank M. *Emergencies in Dental Practice: Prevention and Treatment.* 3rd ed. Philadelphia: Saunders, 1979.

Miller, Glenn A. "Syncope." *Dental Clinics of North American 26* (January 1982).

REVIEW QUESTIONS

MULTIPLE CHOICE

1. The main cause of vasodepressor syncope is:
   a. hunger
   b. stress
   c. excitement
   d. overactivity

2. Which of the following conditions would be considered a psychogenic factor of vasodepressor syncope?
   1. hunger
   2. fear
   3. pain
   4. poor health
      a. 1, 2, 3
      b. 1, 2
      c. 2, 3
      d. 3, 4

3. During which stage of vasodepressor syncope would the patient complain of being dizzy and hot?
   a. syncope
   b. presyncope
   c. a and b
   d. none of the above

4. Which of the following is a sign of the syncope stage?
   1. cold sweat
   2. nausea
   3. dilated pupils
   4. dizziness
      a. 2, 4
      b. 1, 3
      c. 3
      d. 1

5. Placing a patient in the supine position with the feet elevated is known as the _____ position.
   a. Trendelenburg
   b. prone
   c. recovery
   d. syncope

6. In most cases the easiest way to open the airway is the:
   a. jaw-thrust method
   b. head-tilt/chin-lift method
   c. jaw-lift method
   d. none of the above

7. The purpose of the ammonia capsule is to:
   a. burn the nasal passages
   b. stimulate breathing
   c. provide 100 percent oxygen
   d. none of the above

8. The best way to prevent vasodepressor syncope is to:
   a. reduce stress in the office
   b. never see patients with a history of vasodepressor syncope
   c. keep the patient in the Trendelenburg position throughout the entire procedure
   d. all the above

FILL-IN

9. List the signs and symptoms of vasodepressor syncope.
10. List, in order, the treatment for vasodepressor syncope.

TRUE OR FALSE

T 1. Vasodepressor syncope is a life-threatening emergency.
T 2. Once a patient has experienced vasodepressor syncope, he is a likely candidate for it to recur.
F 3. Nonpsychogenic factors are the most common cause of vasodepressor syncope in the dental office.

F   4. Vasodepressor syncope is a loss of consciousness due to an increase in the flow of blood to the brain.

T   5. Fear is a good example of a psychogenic factor causing vasodepressor syncope.

T   6. During presyncope there is a decrease in blood pressure and an increase in pulse rate.

F   7. A good treatment for syncope is to have the patient place the head between the knees.

F   8. Since the patient is unconscious, it is not important for the dental team to remain calm while treating vasodepressor syncope.

T   9. If presyncope is recognized and treated properly most instances of vasodepressor syncope can be prevented.

F   10. The patient may leave the office immediately after recovering from vasodepressor syncope.

■ CASE STUDY

Pauline Peters, 32, in good general health and six months pregnant, has come to the dental office because she has had some pain in the maxillary right central. While waiting for the dentist to come into the operatory, she complains of feeling hot and a little dizzy. A few minutes later she loses consciousness. The auxiliary assumes the patient is suffering from vasodepressor syncope. She places the patient in the Trendelenburg position, administers oxygen, and passes an ammonia capsule underneath the patient's nose.

QUESTIONS

1. What should the auxiliary have done when the patient first began to complain of being hot and dizzy?
2. Why should Pauline Peters not have been placed in the Trendelenburg position?
3. What position should this patient have been placed in?
4. What important treatment step did the auxiliary omit? *vital signs*

4

Airway Obstruction

KEY TERMS

Abdominal thrusts
Asphyxiation
Aspirating
Cyanotic

Dental dam
Heimlich maneuver
Trachea
Tracheotomy

OBJECTIVES

Upon completion of this chapter, the student will be able to:

- Explain several causes of airway obstruction in the dental office
- Explain several ways to prevent airway obstruction in the dental office
- Identify the anatomy of the airway
- Explain the differences between the various types of airway obstructions
- Define the Heimlich maneuver
- Demonstrate the Heimlich maneuver
- Demonstrate manual thrusts
- Demonstrate chest thrusts
- Demonstrate finger sweeps
- Explain the use of the Heimlich on infants

- Explain the use of the Heimlich on children
- Explain the use of the Heimlich on pregnant patients
- Explain the use of the Heimlich on obese patients
- Explain the use of the cricothyrotomy
- Demonstrate how to perform the Heimlich on oneself

Every aspect of the human body depends on the availability of adequate oxygen to function properly. Depriving the body of oxygen for even a few minutes can lead to irreversible brain damage and ultimately to death. It is therefore of utmost importance to recognize and treat airway obstruction both quickly and correctly. Airway obstruction is not selective: young and old alike can be victims.

DENTAL HAZARDS

The dental office is a perfect setting for an airway obstruction to occur. The development of sit-down dentistry, which places the patient in the reclining position, has increased the incidence of dental patients **aspirating** objects into the airway. Practically every aspect of dentistry requires that some object be placed into or taken out of the patient's mouth. These objects, when coated with saliva or blood, can easily slip out of the dentist's or auxiliary's hands and cause an obstruction in the patient. Some items that may be aspirated and produce obstructions (see Emergency Basics) include tooth fragments or whole teeth, amalgam, prosthetic devices, crowns, impression materials, gauze, and cotton rolls.

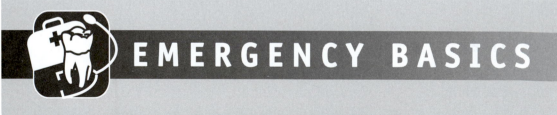

EMERGENCY BASICS

CAUSES OF AIRWAY OBSTRUCTION IN THE DENTAL OFFICE

Cause	Prevention
Extracted teeth	Throat pack
Amalgam	Dental dam and suction
Dental dam clamp	Ligature placed on clamp
Crowns	Throat pack
Impression material	Keep patient positioned upright
Broken burs	Dental dam

The use of certain protective devices such as the **dental dam** or throat packs helps prevent a number of possible airway obstructions. However, some methods of treatment make it impossible to use these devices; in these cases extra precautions must be taken. The auxiliary should be very assertive with the oral evacuator and have the cotton pliers available to retrieve any dropped object.

If an object is dropped, it is extremely important to remain calm to keep the patient from overreacting. Most of the time the patient's gag reflex causes her to cough the object back into the mouth where it can be removed.

ANATOMY OF THE AIRWAY

Most airway obstructions dental personnel encounter occur in the upper airway. To know what occurs during an obstruction, it is important to understand the anatomy of the upper airway. The mouth and nose empty into a common passage called the pharynx, or throat. At the pharynx two passages extend downward. The first passage is the **trachea**, commonly called the windpipe. The trachea is the largest passage, located in the front of the throat, and carries air from the pharynx into the lungs. The second passage is the esophagus, located behind the trachea, which carries solids and liquids from the mouth to the stomach.

When food is swallowed, it is kept out of the trachea by the epiglottis, a flap that covers the opening of the trachea whenever food approaches. In some cases food or other objects get past the epiglottis and pass into the trachea. The majority of the time the patient coughs and the object is removed. However, in some instances the object becomes lodged in the trachea, and an airway obstruction occurs. The upper-airway anatomy is completed by the larynx, or voice box. (The lower airway consists of the bronchi, alveoli, and lungs.)

TYPES OF AIRWAY OBSTRUCTIONS

Airway obstructions can result from a number of situations such as trauma, foreign objects, secretions, burns, or tumors. No matter what the cause, several different types of airway obstructions may occur.

A partial airway obstruction occurs when the airway is not completely blocked. In this situation some air gets through to the lungs. A partial obstruction can be one with adequate air exchange or one with inadequate air exchange. A person suffering from a partial obstruction with adequate air exchange coughs forcibly. This victim is able to talk and may try to explain that the object "went down the wrong way." Such a person is usually not in serious trouble.

The person suffering from a partial obstruction with inadequate air exchange is certainly in danger. She does not cough, although she may make a crowing noise that is a result of the air passing over the lodged object. As the episode progresses, the victim may show signs of cyanosis around the mouth because of the lack of oxygen. The main problem with this situation is that it can easily become a complete airway obstruction. This patient may not be receiving enough oxygen to sustain life and may lose consciousness, suffer brain damage, or die.

The complete airway obstruction is the most life-threatening. The individual suffering from this condition is not able to make any noise but may exhibit the universal distress signal, clutching the throat with the hands (Figure 4-1). The patient usually panics very quickly and may run from the area. If the obstruction is not removed, the patient loses consciousness quickly. If the oxygen is lacking for about four to six minutes, irreversible brain damage can occur, and ultimately, if the object is not removed, the patient will die.

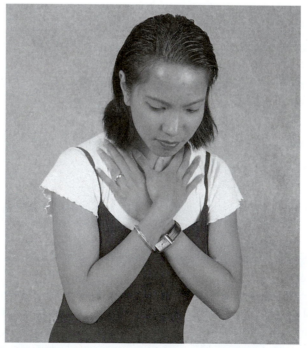

Figure 4-1 Universal distress signal

THE HEIMLICH MANEUVER

Throughout history people have had their own remedies for choking; in most cases the treatments were unsuccessful. Dr. Heimlich developed a technique for relieving airway obstructions that has become known as the **Heimlich maneuver** and consists of a series of manual thrusts. The Heimlich maneuver makes use of the air that remains in the victim's lungs. The pressure placed on the abdomen during manual thrusts causes an elevation of the diphragm, which increases pressure on the lungs and causes an explosive force of air to be released and hopefully to clear the trachea. Since the invention of the Heimlich maneuver, there has been a great deal of controversy over its use. Injuries such as fractured ribs have been noted as a result of the maneuver performed incorrectly. However, the Heimlich maneuver has been found to be successful unless the object cannot be removed, the maneuver is done incorrectly, or too much time elapsed before the technique was started.

Classifications of Airway Obstructions

As mentioned earlier, there are several different degrees of airway obstruction, and, accordingly, different techniques to treat them.

Partial Obstruction with Adequate Air Exchange

This patient coughs forcibly. The only treatment that should be necessary is encouragement to cough. Most of the time, the object is expelled.

Partial Obstruction with Inadequate Air Exchange

This patient is in a potentially life threatening situation, since the obstruction is so great as to prevent the patient from receiving adequate oxygen. This patient should be treated as if suffering from a complete airway obstruction.

Complete Airway Obstruction

A person suffering from a complete airway obstruction cannot breathe, cannot make any sound, becomes extremely pale and **cyanotic**, and may die from **asphyxiation** in approximately four to five minutes. It is of utmost importance that this condition be diagnosed and treated immediately. In this situation the best treatment the auxiliary can provide is the Heimlich maneuver plus additional steps. The maneuver consists of: (1) manual thrusts and (2) finger sweeps (unconscious patient only).

Technique

Manual thrusts may be administered as **abdominal thrusts** or chest thrusts. Both techniques are successful; the patient and the circumstances determine which technique should be used. Chest thrusts are used most often on the pregnant patient or the patient who is extremely obese. The abdominal thrust may be performed on any other patient.

Abdominal Thrust

■ *Conscious Patient*

1. Stand behind the patient.
2. Wrap your arms around the patient.
3. Make a fist with one of your hands.
4. Place the thumb of the fist against the patient's abdomen halfway between the navel and the rib cage.
5. Cover the fist with your other hand.
6. Push the fist quickly four times into the abdomen with an inward and upward motion. (See Figure 4-2).

■ *Unconscious Patient*

1. Place the patient in a supine position.
2. Straddle the patient, facing toward the patient's head. If the patient is small you may stand or kneel alongside.
3. Place the heel of one hand on the patient's abdomen.
4. Place the other hand on top of the first hand and interlock the fingers.
5. Push the heel of the hand rapidly inward and upward four times into the abdomen. (See Figure 4-3).

Chest Thrust

■ *Conscious Patient*

1. Stand behind the patient.
2. Wrap your arms around the patient.
3. Make a fist with one hand.
4. Place the thumb of the fist against the patient's lower sternum. When administering chest thrusts, it is important not to place the hands over the xiphoid process, which could break and cause a laceration of the liver.

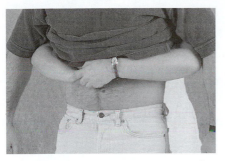

Figure 4-2 Abdominal thrusts on a conscious victim

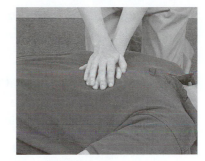

Figure 4-3 Abdominal thrusts on an unconscious victim

5. Place the other hand over the fist.
6. Administer four quick thrusts.

■ *Unconscious Patient*

1. Place the patient in the supine position.
2. Position yourself either beside or straddling the patient.
3. Place the heel of one hand on the patient's lower sternum. Be sure not to place the hand on the xiphoid process.
4. Place the other hand on top of the first and interlock the fingers.
5. Administer four quick downward chest thrusts.

Finger Sweeps

Finger sweeps consist of wiping the patient's oral cavity with the fingers to discover if the obstruction can be reached with your fingers. The procedure is performed only on the unconscious patient. Finger sweeps can be very effective, although they must be used with caution. Care must be taken not to force the object farther down the throat and create a more complete obstruction. Objects should be removed with the fingers only if they are well into the oral cavity and can be easily reached with the fingers.

1. Open the patient's mouth.
2. Use the index and middle fingers.
3. Place the fingers at the corner of the mouth and, using a hooking motion, sweep across the inside of the mouth to the other side.
4. Perform two finger sweeps.

Order of Procedure: Complete Obstruction

■ *Conscious Patient*

1. Stand behind the patient.
2. Administer four manual thrusts.
3. Repeat until the object is removed or the patient loses consciousness.

■ *Unconscious Patient*

1. Place the patient in the supine position.
2. Open the airway.
3. Attempt to ventilate the patient using mouth-to-mouth technique.
4. If you are unable to get air into the patient's lungs, reopen the airway and attempt to ventilate again.
5. Administer four manual thrusts.
6. Make two finger sweeps.
7. Repeat the sequence until the object is removed or surgical intervention is performed by trained personnel.

Note: It is important to continue the Heimlich maneuver even when the patient loses consciousness because the muscles that were constricting and holding the object in place while the patient was conscious may relax during unconsciousness and allow the object to be removed.

HEIMLICH MANEUVER ON INFANTS AND CHILDREN

Choking is the leading cause of death of infants less than one year of age. When administering the Heimlich maneuver on an infant in or out of the dental office, several modifications in technique must be performed. The infant suffering from a complete airway obstruction does not make any sound, turns pale and cyanotic, and collapses due to asphyxiation.

Treatment

■ *Conscious Infant*

1. Place the infant supine on your lap or on a firm surface, depending on your own size.
2. Place the tips of your index and middle fingers halfway between the infant's navel and rib cage.

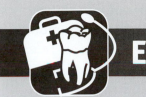

EMERGENCY BASICS

Summary of Treatment for Airway Obstruction

Partial obstruction—adequate air exchange

1. Encourage the patient to cough

Partial obstruction—inadequate air exchange

1. Treat the condition as if the patient was suffering from a complete obstruction

Complete airway obstruction

Conscious

1. Four manual thrusts
2. Repeat sequence until object is dislodged or patient loses consciousness

Unconscious

1. Open airway
2. Attempt to ventilate
3. In unable, reposition airway
4. Attempt to ventilate
5. Four manual thrusts
6. Two finger sweeps
7. Repeat sequence

3. Press inward and upward into the abdomen with four quick movements.
4. If the object is not removed after the four manual thrusts, turn the infant onto its stomach with the head lower than the feet and apply four back blows between the shoulder blades.
5. Repeat the sequence until the infant recovers or loses consciousness.

■ *Unonscious Infant*

1. Place the infant supine on your lap or on a hard surface, depending on your own size.
2. Open the airway.
3. Attempt to ventilate.
4. If no response, reopen the airway.
5. Attempt to ventilate.
6. Place the tips of your index and middle fingers halfway between the infant's navel and rib cage.
7. Press inward and upward into the abdomen with four quick movements.
8. Turn the infant onto its stomach with the head lower than the feet and apply four back blows between the shoulder blades.
9. Using the index finger, perform two finger sweeps if the object is visible in the infant's mouth.
10. Repeat the sequence until the infant recovers or surgical intervention is performed by trained personnel.

On a child (one through eight years of age), the Heimlich maneuver may be performed the same as on an adult, although it is necessary to reduce the force of all actions. When the child or infant recovers, whether in or out of the dental office, she should be chekced by a physician to make sure no additional damage has occurred.

Oral Piercing

Body piercing has become a more prevalent form of body art in today's society. Oral piercing, which may involve the tongue, lips, uvula, or a combination of sites, has been implicated in several adverse oral conditions.

Examples of these conditions may include:
■ gingival injury or recession
■ damage to teeth or restorations
■ interference with speech or chewing and swallowing
■ scar tissue formation
■ prolonged bleeding
■ severe infection

A true emergency related to oral piercing might present itself in the form of an airway obstruction. It is possible that the jewelry may become dislodged and pass into the airway. When dental personnel are providing treatment for a patient who has some form of oral piercing they should take precautions to avoid dislodging the jewelry.

Because of the potential for various related complications, the American Dental Association opposes the practice of oral piercing.

SPECIAL PATIENTS

Some patients other than children and infants may sometimes present problems that require you to make adjustments in the way you perform the Heimlich maneuver.

The first case is the pregnant patient. Not only do you not want to take the chance of damaging the unborn child by applying abdominal thrusts, but the size of the patient sometimes makes it physically impossible to perform the maneuver. Whenever this kind of patient is suffering from an airway obstruction, the best method of treatment is to perform the Heimlich maneuver exactly as previously stated, except to employ chest thrusts in place of abdominal thrusts. This is the only major adjustment that should be necessary on the pregnant patient. Remember, however, that when the mother is deprived of oxygen, the baby is also deprived. All steps should be taken immediately to restore oxygen to this patient.

The second type of patient who may present specific problems is the extremely obese one. The size of this patient may prevent you from being able to perform any type of manual thrusts when standing behind the patient because you may not be able to wrap your arms completely around the body. In such cases all manual thrusts must be performed from the front. To make these steps easier to perform, it is best to have the patient either lying down or seated.

Special circumstances require special actions. The important thing to remember is that the patient can survive for only a very short period of time without oxygen, and the main goal is to do whatever is necessary to clear the obstruction and get oxygen to the patient.

CRICOTHYROTOMY

No matter how well the Heimlich maneuver is performed, there are some situations in which is is not successful. If such a situation arises, it may be necessary to use surgical intervention.

The method of choice was formerly a **tracheotomy**. However, the area where a tracheotomy must be performed is very close to several large sources of blood and nerve supplies. It is very easy to cause severe problems with this technique even when performed in the best of circumstances, to say nothing of an emergency situation. As a result, the cricothyrotomy has replaced the tracheotomy as the treatment of choice when an emergency airway must be provided.

Any type of surgical airway intervention should be used only by someone trained in its use and then only as a last resort.

A cricothyrotomy is performed as follows:

1. Locate the cricothyroid membrane by placing the finger on the Adam's apple and sliding downward toward the feet until you feel a slight indented area. This is the cricothyroid membrane.
2. Using a sharp object, preferably a scalpel, make an incision in this area, then widen the incision. There will be little bleeding because there are no major blood vessels in this area.
3. The opening must be maintained. Place an item such as a holder for a ballpiont ben, a suction tip, or your finger into the incision to keep the airway open. If necessary, artificial respiration may be administered through this temporary air space.

A modification of this technique is use of the cricothyrotomy needle (Figure 4-4). Practially every emergency kit contains such an item. The needle has a very large diameter, which permits air to pass through. The method detailed above would be used with one exception: instead of making an incision, the needle would be inserted into the cricothyroid membrane.

PERFORMING THE HEIMLICH ON YOURSELF

Manual thrusts may be performed on yourself if you are choking and no help is available.

1. Place your hands in the position described for abdominal thrusts, and press.
2. Place yourself against the banister of a stairway, corner of a sink, or arm of a chair and press quickly against it. These techniques are by no means as effective as the full Heimlich maneuver but may prove effective when no other means of help is available.

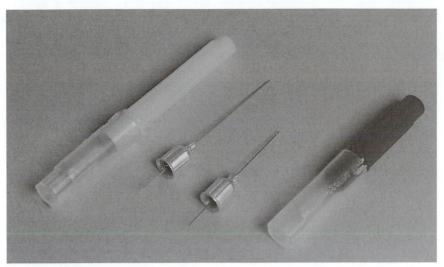

Figure 4-4 Cricothyrotomy needle in sterile case

SUMMARY

An airway obstruction can occur at any time to any patient. Brain damage or death can occur very quickly as a result of an airway obstruction. It is therefore of utmost importance that the dental auxiliary recognize the condition quickly and treat it effectively.

REFERENCES

"Airway Obstruction: Guidelines for Management." *Hospital Medicine* (June 1983).

Grant, Harvey, and Robert Murray. *Emergency Care*. 2nd ed. Bowie, Md.: Robert J. Brady Co., 1978.

Guildner, Charles Wayne. "Airway Obstructed by Foreign Material: The Heimlich Maneuver." *Journal of American Clinical Emergency Physicians 5* (September 1976).

Levine, Irene. "Update on Upper Airway Management." *Patient Care* (September 15, 1978).

Malamed, Stanley F. *Handbook of Medical Emergencies in the Dental Office*. 2nd ed. St. Louis: Mosby, 1982.

McCarthy, Frank M. *Medical Emergencies in Dentistry: An Abridged Edition*. 3rd ed. Philadelphia: Saunders, 1982.

Oppenheimer, Peter R. "Airway Instantly." *Journal of the American Medical Association 230* (October 7, 1974).

Pellegrino R., et al. "Assessing the reversibility of airway obstruction." *Chest*, Dec. 1998.

Redding, Joseph S. "The Choking Controversy: Critique of Evidence on the Heimlich Maneuver." *Critical Care Medicine 7* (October 1979).

Safar, Peter. "Recognition and Management of Airway Obstruction." *Journal of the American Medical Association 208* (May 12, 1969).

Siegel, Elliot B., and Arthur H. Friedlander. "Emergency Treatment of Foreign Bodies Lodged in the Trachea." *General Dentistry* (September-October 1976).

"Standards and Guidelines for Cardiopulmonary Resuscitation and Emergency Cardiac Care." *Journal of the American Medical Association* (June 1986).

Thompson, Sharon W. "How to Use the Heimlich Maneuver on Choking Infants and Children." *Pediatric Nursing* (Janurary-February 1983).

REVIEW QUESTIONS

MULTIPLE CHOICE

1. The trachea is commonly known as the:
   a. voice box
   b. throat
   c. windpipe
   d. none of the above

2. Which of the follow is true concerning a partial obstruction with inadequate air exchange?
   1. patient may exhibit a crowing sound
   2. should be treated as a complete obstruction
   3. is not a serious condition
   4. patient may be cyanotic
      a. 1, 2, 3, 4
      b. 1, 2, 3
      c. 2, 3, 4
      d. 1, 2, 4

3. What should be the treatment for a patient suffering from a partial obstruction with adequate air exchange?
    a. encourage coughing
    b. administer two finger sweeps
    c. use the full Heimlich
    d. use manual thrusts only

4. Which of the following is true concerning finger sweeps?
    a. Administer finger sweeps only to infants
    b. Finger sweeps are performed only on unconscious victims.
    c. Use two fingers to perform finger sweeps.
    d. b and c

5. It would be best to use chest thrusts on the:
    a. pregnant patient
    b. tall patient
    c. unconscious patient
    d. all the above

6. The universal distress signal is indicated by:
    a. placing the palm of the hand over the mouth
    b. clutching the throat with both hands
    c. covering the eyes with the palms of both hands
    d. none of the above

7. Which of the following techniques is performed only on the unconscious patient?
    1. chest thrusts
    2. finger sweeps
    3. artificial respirations
    4. manual thrusts
        a. 1, 2
        b. 2, 3, 4
        c. 2, 3
        d. 3, 4

8. The tips of the index and middle fingers are used to administer manual thrusts on:
   a. elderly patients
   b. obese patients
   c. pregnant patients
   d. infants

9. What is the most accepted surgical technique for relieving an airway obstruction?
   a. cricothyrotomy
   b. tracheotomy
   c. laryngectomy
   d. none of the above

10. Abdominal thrusts should be administered:
    a. over the diaphragm
    b. over the lower sternum
    c. between the sternum and diaphragm
    d. between the navel and rib cage

TRUE OR FALSE

T 1. Brain damage can occur as a result of a lack of oxygen in as little as four to six minutes.

T 2. The use of the rubber dam may help prevent some airway obstructions.

F 3. It is best to perform manual thrusts while standing in front of the patient.

F 4. The Heimlich maneuver is usually not successful when performed on infants or children.

F 5. The Heimlich maneuver should be stopped once a patient loses consciousness.

T 6. The universal distress signal consists of the victim's clutching the throat with the hands.

F 7. The unconscious patient should be placed in the upright position before administering the Heimlich.

T 8. Chest thrusts are best performed on obese and pregnant patients.

9. Finger sweeps performed incorrectly can force the foreign object back into the victim's throat.

F 10. You should attempt to ventilate a conscious and unconscious patient.

■ CASE STUDY

Robert Jackson, 16 and in good health, has come to the dental office to have a crown cemented on number 30. During the try-in the crown slips from the dentist's hand and goes down the patient's throat. The patient begins to gasp and make a crowing sound. The dental team gets the patient out of the chair and begins to perform the Heimlich. After two sequences, the object is expelled and the patient recovers.

QUESTIONS

1. What type of obstruction is the patient experiencing?
2. What could have been done to prevent this situation from occurring?
3. Explain the steps, in the correct order, of the procedure that would be performed on this patient.

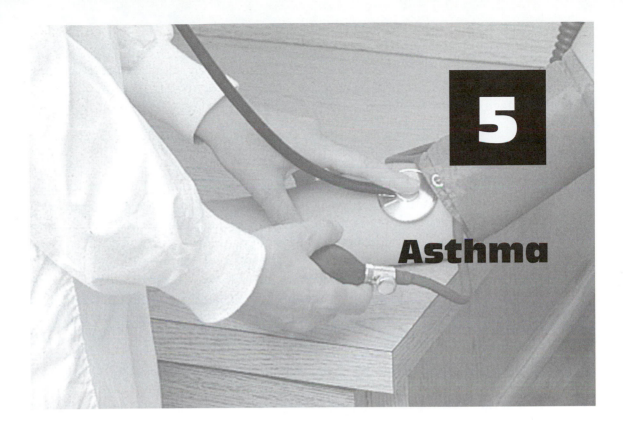

5

Asthma

KEY TERMS

Allergen
Bronchodilator
Epinephrine
Extrinsic asthma

Intrinsic asthma
Status asthmaticus
Tracheobronchial tree

OBJECTIVES

Upon completion of this chapter the student will be able to:

- Define asthma
- Explain two of the causes of asthma
- Describe the signs and symptoms of asthma
- Describe the treatment provided for an asthma attack

Diseases or problems associated with the respiratory system such as asthma, bronchitis, or emphysema may create emergency situations. An asthma attack is one example of a respiratory emergency commonly seen in the dental setting.

Asthma is an affliction of the respiratory tract that can affect all aspects of the **tracheobronchial tree**: trachea, bronchi, and bronchioles. The type of asthma as well as its severity determine what areas of the tracheobronchial tree are involved. Asthma can cause death, but today death from asthma is a rare occurrence. Asthma affects a large percentage of the population and is not selective as to race, sex, or age.

TYPES

Asthma can be divided into different categories. The first is **extrinsic asthma**, or allergic asthma. This type of asthma is reported most often in children and young adults. Episodes of extrinsic asthma usually result from exposure to an **allergen** such as dust, pollen, animals, and certain foods and many other substances. Most patients are aware of the types of allergens that trigger their asthma attacks and try to avoid them. (If the allergens are not known, they can be determined by a physician performing allergy tests.) The dental team should also be aware of any specific allergens that trigger a patient's asthma, making it possible to avoid exposing the patient to them while the patient is in the office.

The patient usually does not exhibit any signs or symptoms of asthma between attacks. Furthermore, extrinsic asthma usually responds well to medication and *may* be outgrown.

The second type of asthma is **intrinsic asthma**, or infectious asthma, most often seen in patients over thirty-five. Intrinsic asthma usually occurs as a result of some type of bronchial infection. Unlike the extrinsic asthma patient, this patient may exhibit a chronic cough with sputum production between attacks.

The most severe form of asthma is **status asthmaticus**, which can occur in any type of asthma. It will not respond to normal drug therapy and will cause death if not treated promptly.

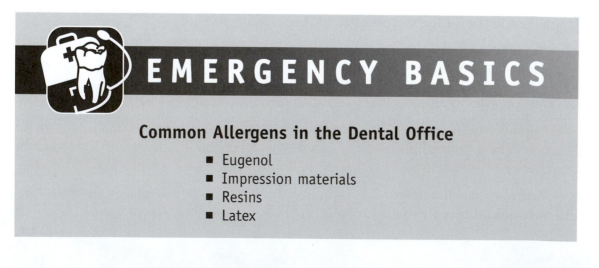

EMERGENCY BASICS

Common Allergens in the Dental Office

- Eugenol
- Impression materials
- Resins
- Latex

The patient may experience extrinsic or intrinsic asthma independently or, sometimes, a combination of the two.

CAUSES

Asthma attacks can be triggered by an almost endless number of causes, both known and unknown. As previously mentioned, exposure to a particular allergen can cause an attack. Anxiety or emotional upset is definitely known to be a factor in triggering asthma attacks—and is the main cause of asthma attacks in the dental office. Some children experience an asthma attack immediately upon entering the dental operatory, one that ends as soon as the child is removed from the operatory. It is extremely important for the dental staff to do everything possible to prevent emotional upsets, including the following measures.

1. Do not keep the patient waiting for an extended period.
2. Explain and demonstrate the procedures and equipment.
3. Do not use threatening terminology such as drill, hurt, and shot.

SYMPTOMS

An asthma attack may occur suddenly without any warning or slowly over an extended period.

When dealing with an asthma patient in an emergency situation, you must first distinguish between asthma and an airway obstruction. If there is confusion, listen to the sounds the patient is making. With airway obstruction, you may hear a stridor—a constant-pitch musical sound during inspirations. With asthma, a wheezing sound heard during expirations is characteristic. In addition, an easy way to determine that the patient is suffering from an asthma attack is to read the health history. If a patient has indicated a history of asthma and then exhibits the signs and symptoms, the attack should be treated as asthma.

During an asthma attack, the bronchioles become narrowed due to contractions of the smooth muscles, and there is an overproduction of mucus. As a result, the air passages are restricted, breathing becomes difficult, and the patient seems to be struggling for air. With asthma, exhaling is the most difficult part of breathing, although most of the time the patient feels as if inhaling is the most difficult.

The patient suffering from an asthma attack may be sweating and coughing, and may appear to be very nervous. The nervousness occurs as a result of the patient's inability to breathe normally. The patient may also complain of a severe tightness in the chest.

During an attack, it is common for blood pressure and pulse to increase slightly. However, in some cases these vital signs may remain close to the baseline readings.

The duration of an asthma attack varies from patient to patient. If left untreated, it may continue anywhere from a few minutes to several hours. The patient usually experiences a severe coughing attack and expectorates a large bolus of mucus immediately before the attack terminates. On the other hand, if the patient is treated immediately with a **bronchodilator**, the attack usually ends within a few seconds.

Status asthmaticus, as already noted, is the most severe form of asthma. It may begin like any other asthma attack but will not respond to any type of treatment or medication, and the patient therefore experiences one continuous asthma attack. The situation may continue for days. This person is in a life-threatening situation and should be in the hospital.

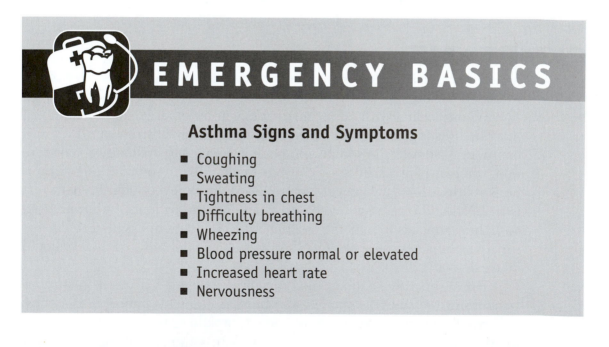

EMERGENCY BASICS

Asthma Signs and Symptoms

- Coughing
- Sweating
- Tightness in chest
- Difficulty breathing
- Wheezing
- Blood pressure normal or elevated
- Increased heart rate
- Nervousness

TREATMENT

Once it has been determined that the patient is suffering from an asthma attack, prompt treatment should be administered.

1. Stop all dental treatment. Be sure to remove all materials and instruments from the patient's mouth. The patient will be breathing forcibly, so be sure there are no cotton rolls or other small items left in the mouth for the patient to inhale.
2. Position the patient. Raise the patient upright; he will be struggling for air and will breathe easier if seated upright.
3. Use a bronchodilator. The patient's health history will state whether he suffers from asthma. On reading this information, the dental auxiliary should ask if the patient is carrying a bronchodilator (Figure 5-1). The bronchodilator is an aerosol medication that usually includes **epinephrine** and is used to treat the attack. It relaxes the bronchioles, which makes it easier for the patient to breathe. The patient's bronchodilator should be placed within easy reach in case an attack occurs. If the attack takes place, allow the patient to administer his bronchodilator: patients know what their usual dose involves.
4. Administer oxygen. Administer four to six liters of oxygen per minute by a full-face mask or nasal canula, if one is available. Be careful not to frighten the patient when you apply the face mask. Asthma patients are struggling for air and may get a feeling of suffocation from the oxygen

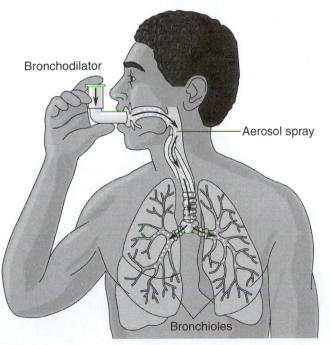

Figure 5-1 Use of a bronchodilator

EMERGENCY BASICS

Treatment for Asthma

1. Stop dental treatment
2. Position patient
3. Administer bronchodilator
4. Administer oxygen
5. Administer epinephrine IV
6. Summon medical help

mask. Solve this problem by allowing the patient to hold the mask himself.

5. If the bronchodilator does not relieve the attack, it may be necessary for the dentist to administer epinephrine or another drug intravenously. The auxiliary should set up the IV according to the dentist's instructions.

6. If the steps listed above are not successful, call for medical assistance. Remember, if all treatment is unsuccessful, the patient may be suffering from status asthmaticus and should be hospitalized as soon as possible.

SUMMARY

Asthma attacks in the dental office are most often triggered by anxiety. Therefore it is extremely important to try to keep all patients calm, especially the asthma patient. If an asthma attack does occur, try to calm the patient while administering prompt, efficient treatment.

REFERENCES

Alcock SM, et al. "Symptoms and pulmonary function in asthma." *Respir Med*, June 1998.

Carson, Ruth. "Asthma: How to Live with It." Public Affairs Pamphlet No. 437.

Grant, Harvey, and Robert Murray. *Emergency Care*. 2nd ed. Bowie, Maryland: Robert J. Brady Co., 1978.

Malamed, Stanley F. *Handbook of Medical Emergencies in the Dental Office*. 2nd ed. St. Louis: Mosby, 1982.

Saltman, Jules. "Asthma Episodes and Treatment." Public Affairs Pamphlet No. 608.

Sanders, Frank. "A Basic Approach to Asthma." *Consultant* (February 1980).

"The Treatment of Asthma." *The New England Journal of Medicine 298* (February 16, 1978).

Watanabe T., et al. "Decrease in emergency room or urgent care visits due to management of bronchial asthma inpatients and outpatient with pharmaceutical services." *J Clin Pharm Ther.*, August 1998.

REVIEW QUESTIONS

MULTIPLE CHOICE

1. What type of asthma is considered the most life-threatening?
   a. status asthmaticus
   b. intrinsic asthma
   c. extrinsic asthma
   d. infectious asthma

2. Which of the following is not a sign or symptom of asthma?
   a. wheezing
   b. tightness in the chest
   c. coughing
   d. stridor

3. What type of asthma is usually reported in young children?
   a. extrinsic
   b. infectious
   c. intrinsic
   d. none of the above

4. What type of asthma usually occurs as a result of a bronchial infection?
   a. status asthmaticus
   b. extrinsic asthma
   c. allergic asthma
   (d.) none of the above

5. A/An _____ may be administered by the patient to relieve her asthma.
   a. injection
   (b.) bronchodilator
   c. IV
   d. tablet

TRUE OR FALSE

T 1. An asthma attack may occur suddenly or over a long period of time.
F 2. Oxygen should not be administered to the asthma patient.
T 3. A patient suffering from status asthmaticus should be hospitalized as soon as possible.
F 4. Asthma only begins in young children.
F 5. Today, all causes of asthma are known.

■ CASE STUDY

Bobby Thompson, 10 years old, suffers from extrinsic asthma. He is in the dental office to have two teeth extracted for orthodontic purposes. The dentist is running behind and Bobby has to wait for twenty minutes before he is taken to the operatory. Once there Bobby begins to cough, wheeze, and struggle for air. The dentist, aware of Bobby's condition, sends the auxiliary to the waiting room to get the bronchodilator from Bobby's mother. During this time the dentist stops the treatment and talks calmly to Bobby. Once Bobby administers his bronchodilator, he recovers completely.

QUESTIONS

1. How could keeping Bobby waiting in the waiting room add to the chances of the asthma attack occurring? *Causes anxiety*
2. Where should Bobby's bronchodilator have been placed during the treatment? *In Bobby's pocket*
3. What was the main cause of Bobby's asthma attack? *stress*

6

Hyperventilation

KEY TERMS
Carbon dioxide
Diazepam

OBJECTIVES
Upon completion of this chapter the student will be able to:
- Define hyperventilation
- Describe the signs and symptoms of hyperventilation
- Explain the causes of hyperventilation
- Explain the treatment of hyperventilation
- Describe the best way to prevent hyperventilation

Hyperventilation is an increase in the rate or depth of breathing that results in a change in the blood chemistry and usually occurs as a result of anxiety. The dental office is an anxious setting for most people, which is why hyperventilation is a very common emergency seen there.

CAUSES

The most common cause of hyperventilation is anxiety. Although not as common, hyperventilation may also be caused by certain physical conditions, emotional upset, or stress.

Hyperventilation is not normally encountered in children. It has been stated that hyperventilation occurs most often in patients who hide their feelings and do not admit their fears of dentistry. In such a person, the anxiety builds up within until the patient can no longer control it. Children usually cry or scream when frightened, which expresses their fears and prevents hyperventilation from occurring.

PHYSIOLOGY

Carbon dioxide in the blood automatically triggers the breathing reflex and stimulates respiration. In this way it helps control the breathing process automatically. A person who begins to hyperventilate increases the depth and rate of respirations much like an athlete who has performed strenuous exercise. By increasing respirations, they exhale a large amount of carbon dioxide. In the athlete, the exercised muscles release carbon dioxide into the blood, which replenishes the excess given off by the rapid breathing. Because the dental patient is motionless, however, she has no way of replenishing the carbon dioxide she is exhaling. Therefore she suffers from a lack of carbon dioxide and has problems breathing. When there is a lack of carbon dioxide, the patient must consciously work to inhale and exhale.

Hyperventilation takes place in a cycle. First, the patient becomes very anxious about the dental treatment. This results in the patient beginning to hyperventilate. Next, the patient begins to realize she is having difficulty breathing. This then makes the patient more anxious, which worsens the hyperventilation. This cycle will increase in severity unless someone intervenes. It is of utmost importance for the members of the dental team to recognize the problem, intervene, and attempt to calm the patient.

SIGNS AND SYMPTOMS

A patient first entering the operatory may appear nervous or anxious but usually does not discuss her fear of the dental procedure. The patient begins to breathe deeper and faster. At this point, she usually does not realize there has been a change in breathing pattern. The patient may then complain of a feeling of suffocation and tightness in the chest. As she continues to hyper-

EMERGENCY BASICS

Signs and Symptoms of Hyperventilation

- Nervousness
- Increase in rate of respirations
- Feeling of suffocation
- Tightness in chest
- Dizziness
- Tingling in extremities

ventilate, she may experience a feeling of dizziness. If the syndrome is allowed to continue, tingling may develop in the extremities.

These patients are in respiratory distress, although they will not be cyanotic as in other cases because they are receiving plenty of oxygen. Their lack of carbon dioxide is the problem in this situation.

TREATMENT

Hyperventilation is an emergency situation that can usually be corrected by performing these steps:

1. Once it has been determined that the patient is hyperventilating, stop all dental treatment. Be sure to remove any objects from the patient's mouth.
2. Place the patient in an upright position. The patient is having difficulty breathing and will be more comfortable sitting upright.
3. Attempt to calm the patient, who will be very agitated and will be breathing rapidly. Explain the condition to the patient. Tell the patient to inhale and hold her breath for several seconds before exhaling. This procedure will help increase the level of carbon dioxide.
4. In some cases the patient may be upset, and you will not be able to convince the person to hold her breath for even a second. Therefore you will have to increase the level of carbon dioxide by using other techniques. The easiest method is to have the patient breathe into a paper

EMERGENCY BASICS

Treatment for Hyperventilation

1. Stop dental treatment
2. Position the patient
3. Calm the patient
4. Have the patient breathe into paper bag
5. Administer drug therapy (if needed)

sack. The hyperventilating patient has a sense of suffocation, so be very careful not to startle the patient by placing the bag over the face. Instead, let the patient hold the bag to give her a sense of controlling the situation. Once the bag is in place, instruct the patient to breathe in and out of the bag (Figure 6-1). The patient will be inhaling carbon dioxide, and this will help end the syndrome. Be sure never to use any type of plastic bag.

5. Never administer oxygen to a hyperventilating patient. Remember, this patient already has too much oxygen and too little carbon dioxide.
6. If the patient is experiencing a severe hyperventilation episode, it may be necessary for the dentist to administer a drug to reduce anxiety.

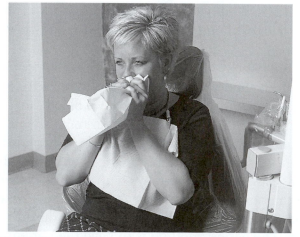

Figure 6-1 Hyperventilating patient breathes into a paper bag

Diazepam (Valium) is usually the drug. If this step is necessary, prepare the drug according to the dentist's instructions.

SUMMARY

Hyperventilation in the dental office usually occurs as a result of anxiety. It is very important for the dental team to determine what caused the person's fears of dentistry. Once this is established, it is easier for the dental team to take steps to alleviate the fears and, hopefully, prevent a hyperventilation episode.

REFERENCES

Dalessio, Donald. "Hyperventilation. The Vapors. Effort Syndrome. Neurasthenia." *Journal of the American Medical Association* (April 1978).

Grant, Harvey, and Robert Murray. *Emergency Care*. 2nd ed. Bowie, Maryland: Robert J. Brady Co., 1978.

Malamed, Stanley F. *Handbook of Medical Emergencies in the Dental Office*. 2nd ed. St. Louis: Mosby, 1982.

REVIEW QUESTIONS

MULTIPLE CHOICE

1. Which of the following groups is most unlikely to experience hyperventilation?
   a. young adults
   b. children
   c. elderly
   d. all the above

2. The patient who hyperventilates is suffering from a lack of:
   a. carbon dioxide
   b. oxygen
   c. nitrogen
   d. hydrogen

3. The most common cause of hyperventilation is:
   a. overexertion
   b. high blood pressure
   c. lack of oxygen
   d. none of the above

4. Which of the following is a sign or symptom of hyperventilation?
   a. nervousness
   b. rapid breathing
   c. feeling of suffocation
   d. all the above

5. What is usually the drug of choice if medication is used to treat the hyperventilating patient?
   a. diazepam
   b. dilantin
   c. epinephrine
   d. none of the above

TRUE OR FALSE

F 1. Hyperventilation is one of the most uncommon emergencies experienced in the dental office.

T 2. Hyperventilation can usually be relieved by having the patient breathe into a plastic bag.

T 3. The rate and depth of respirations increase dramatically in the hyperventilating patient.

T 4. Hyperventilation usually occurs as a result of a lack of carbon dioxide.

F 5. The hyperventilating dental patient should be placed in the supine position.

■ CASE STUDY

Suzanne Mays is a 35-year-old patient in good general health. She has come to the office to have an amalgam placed in tooth number 20. Once seated in the dental chair, Suzanne begins to talk rapidly and clutches the arms of the chair. She admits no fear of the dental procedure but appears to be very nervous, then begins to breathe rapidly and complains of a tightness in the chest and a feeling of suffocation. She is hyperventilating.

QUESTIONS

1. Describe, in order, the type of treatment that should be given to this patient.
2. How could the dental auxiliary prevent this situation from occurring on the patient's next visit?
3. Why should oxygen not be administered in this situation?

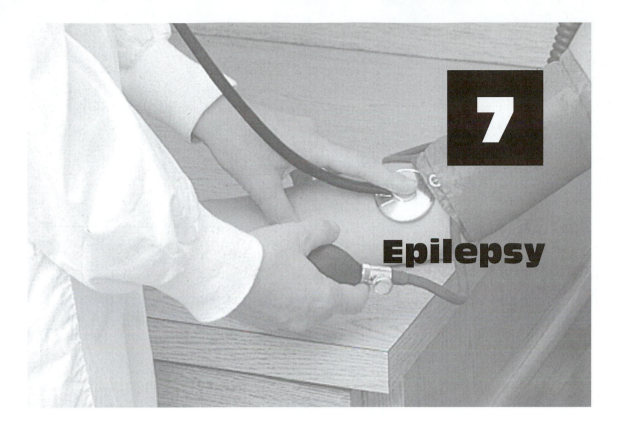

7

Epilepsy

KEY TERMS

Aura
Clonic
Dilantin hyperplasia
Grand mal seizure

Partial seizure
Petit mal seizure
Status epilepticus
Tonic

OBJECTIVES

Upon completion of this chapter the student will be able to:

- Define epilepsy
- Explain some of the causes of epilepsy
- Describe what takes place during a grand mal seizure
- Define an absence seizure
- Define a partial seizure
- Describe status epilepticus
- Explain the treatment of an epiletic seizure
- Describe some possible dental implications of epilepsy
- Explain how some epileptic seizures may be prevented

An epileptic seizure occurs as a result of a sudden discharge of electrical energy somewhere in the central nervous system caused by an imbalance among the neurons of the brain. The area of the brain that is affected determines the type of seizure the epileptic experiences. Epilepsy is a mysterious disease that affects people for a variety of reasons and is not selective as to race, age, or sex.

CAUSES

In the majority of cases the cause of epilepsy is unknown, but in a few types of epilepsy the cause of the disease has been determined. First, an accident, such as a fall or a car accident, that damages the brain can result in the person becoming an epileptic. Epilepsy may also be caused by injury during birth, a severe infection, or a fever high enough to cause damage to the brain. Furthermore, heredity plays a role in the cause of epilepsy. It has been documented that if both parents are epileptics, the chances of their offspring becoming epileptics are greatly increased.

TYPES OF SEIZURES

Epileptic seizures are usually identified by the actions that occur while the seizure is in progress. **Grand mal seizures** are the most common. The grand mal seizure is also known as the tonic/clonic seizure from the body movements the patient makes during the seizure. The grand mal seizure can be divided into three phases: prodromal, convulsive, and postictal.

The first phase is the prodromal phase, which includes the period before the actual seizure occurs. During this period, the patient may experience slight personality changes. These are usually so subtle that they are noticed only by people who are very close to the patient, such as family members. Some patients may experience an **aura** during this phase. The aura may consist of a certain smell, a flash of light, or a certain noise. Auras are usually unique to the individual and occur just before the patient advances to the convulsive phase.

The convulsive phase consists of the actual **tonic** and **clonic** movements. The patient loses consciousness, falls down, and in some instances gives out the epileptic cry. This cry results from the air rushing out of the lungs as the patient loses consciousness. Next, the patient's body stiffens and becomes rigid—the tonic stage. As the patient passes into the clonic stage, the body begins to jerk violently. There may be foaming at the mouth,

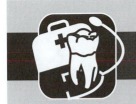

EMERGENCY BASICS

Phases of the Grand Mal Seizure

Prodromal: personality change
aura

Convulsive: tonic movements
clonic movements
sphincter muscle control loss
bladder control loss

Postictal: regaining of consciousness
confusion
deep sleep

caused by air mixing with the blood and saliva. The patient may also not be able to control bladder or sphincter muscles.

The final phase of the grand mal seizure consists of the postictal phase. During this phase, the actual seizure is over, and the patient should slowly begin to regain consciousness. The patient may be confused about what happened or where he is. In addition, he may need to sleep for a while in order to recover.

The second type of seizure is the **petit mal seizure**. It is sometimes called an "absence seizure," which best describes what occurs during the seizure. The patient experiencing an absence seizure loses awareness of the surroundings for a very short time. He may have a blank stare, twitch, or blink rapidly. This type of seizure may come and go without anyone around the patient realizing that he is experiencing a seizure. This type of seizure is seen most often in children and is often misdiagnosed as a behavioral problem in school-age children.

The third type of seizure is the **partial seizure**. This seizure involves only one hemisphere of the brain, so the patient may experience a jerking movement of only one part of the body, such as a leg or arm, rather than convulsive movements of the entire body. In addition, this person may appear to be in a trance-like state and may fidget, pick at clothing, or wander around.

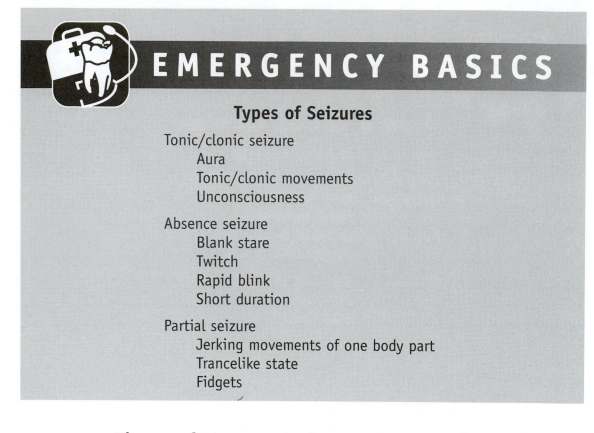

EMERGENCY BASICS

Types of Seizures

Tonic/clonic seizure
- Aura
- Tonic/clonic movements
- Unconsciousness

Absence seizure
- Blank stare
- Twitch
- Rapid blink
- Short duration

Partial seizure
- Jerking movements of one body part
- Trancelike state
- Fidgets

The most dangerous type of seizure is **status epilepticus**, which is extremely dangerous and causes death in 10 percent of cases. During status epilepticus, the patient either experiences one seizure after another or experiences one continuous seizure. The body cannot handle this condition, and the patient is in a life-threatening situation.

TREATMENT

Witnessing an epileptic seizure can be traumatic. When treating an epileptic patient, try to stay calm and remember that the seizure is usually brief, is usually not life-threatening, and requires very little care.

As far as the dental team is concerned, the main method of treatment for an epileptic seizure should be to keep the patient from hurting himself during the actual seizure and to provide supportive help once the seizure is over.

Follow these steps:

1. Remove all dental objects from the patient's mouth.
2. Remove all dental equipment on which the patient may hit and injure himself, but if possible do not move the patient. However, if a patient is in the dental chair and there are certain objects that cannot be moved on which you think the patient may be injured, move the patient to the floor.
3. Remove glasses and loosen tight clothing such as neckties. Dentures or partial dentures should remain in the patient's mouth unless they are causing an airway obstruction.
4. If possible, place a tongue depressor wrapped in adhesive tape between the patient's teeth. This procedure may help keep the patient from biting his tongue. However, it is important to remember that the patient's jaws may clamp together at any moment with enough force to severely injure your finger. Therefore, if the patient's teeth are clenched or there is any difficulty getting the tongue blade in place, omit this procedure.
5. Do not restrain the patient. If you try to restrict the patient from making the convulsive movements, you may injure the patient's muscles or tendons. These movements are so forceful that restraint may injure the patient and possibly even you, if you are hit by a flying arm or leg. The patient need be restricted only to the point of preventing injury, such

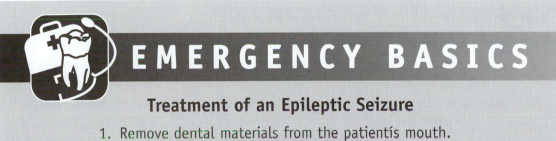

EMERGENCY BASICS

Treatment of an Epileptic Seizure

1. Remove dental materials from the patientís mouth.
2. Remove objects that may injure the patient.
3. Remove glasses and loosen clothing.
4. Place a tongue depressor between the teeth if possible.
5. Do not restrain the patient.
6. Place the patient on one side once the seizure is over.
7. Reassure the patient.
8. Do not give the patient anything to eat or drink.
9. Let the patient recover.

as hitting the head on the floor or injuring extremities on a nearby object.

6. Once the seizure has ended, turn the patient on one side so any secretions are not aspirated. Remember during the entire seizure that an opened airway must be maintained above all else.

7. The patient who begins to regain consciousness needs reassurance and may be confused as to what happened and what day it is. Also, most patients will be embarassed by the episode; you should whatever possible to alleviate this embarrassment.

8. Do not give the patient anything to eat or drink until he is fully alert.

9. The patient should be given plenty of time to rest and recover—some patients go into a deep sleep for several hours. The patient should be placed in an appropriate area and allowed to remain there until fully recovered.

Most epileptic seizures can be treated primarily by letting them run their own course. However, in some cases you should summon medical assistance:

1. If the patient is injured during the seizure
2. If the patient stops breathing and does not recuperate immediately
3. If the seizure seems to pass from one episode right into the next, which would indicate the possibility of status epilepticus

DENTAL IMPLICATIONS OF EPILEPSY

The dental office is a likely setting for the occurrence of an epileptic seizure, just as it is for many other stress-related emergencies. Furthermore, the dental office may have to deal with special situations related to epilepsy.

Dilantin, one of the drugs commonly given to treat epileptics, may produce a condition known as **dilantin hyperplasia**, in which the gingival tissue grows at a rapid rate and in some cases covers the teeth completely. In such extreme cases, the tissue is surgically removed.

Epilepsy may dictate the type of treatment the dentist may perform. For instance, it has been noted that removable appliances have lodged in areas of the sinus during a seizure and not been found until the patient started having sinus-related problems. This suggests that the dentist should consider fixed appliances, if feasible, when treating an epileptic patient with prosthetic devices.

PREVENTION

Most of the cases of epilepsy are still unknown, and in these circumstances it is impossible to prevent people from becoming epileptic. However, in most cases it is possible to control the epilepsy and prevent seizures by administering an anticonvulsant, the most common of which is dilantin, as noted above. An anticonvulsant cannot cure epilepsy, but it can control the seizures in about 75 percent of patients.

If an epileptic seizure takes place in the dental office, it is important to try to remember what happened before the attack occurred; this may help determine what triggered the seizure. For example, was a material used that had a distinct odor, or an instrument that emitted a particular sound? By making this determination, it may be possible to prevent future seizures from occurring in the dental office.

It has been noted that an epileptic seizure may be triggered in some patients by an extremely stressful situation, and to many people the dental office provides just this type of situation. It is, therefore, extremely important to try to eliminate as much stress as possible. There are several ways to achieve this, including:

1. Show and demonstrate the use of all equipment in the office.
2. Do not keep the patient waiting in the reception area.
3. In some cases, premedicate the patient. This step may require a consultation with the patient's physician.

SUMMARY

Epilepsy is a very mysterious and frightening disease. However, by being aware of what is taking place during a seizure, members of the dental team can learn to handle the situation quickly and efficiently.

REFERENCES

Dreifuss, Fritz E., Brian B. Gallagher, Ilo E. Lepik, and A. David Rothner. "Keeping Epilepsy Under Control." *Patient Care* (October 15, 1983).

Dreifuss, Fritz E. "Intervening to Stop Status Epilepticus." *Patient Care* (October 15, 1983).

Dreifuss, Fritz E. "Helping Your Patient Live with Epilepsy." *Patient Care* (September 15, 1983).

Edmeads, John. "Terminating Seizures." *Emergency Medicine* (November 30, 1982).

Giovannitti, Joseph A. "Aspiration of a Partial Denture During an Epileptic Seizure." *Journal of the American Dental Association. 112* (May 1980).

Livingston, Samuel, and Lydia L. Pauli. "Guideposts to Managing Epileptic Patients." *Consultants* (April 1979).

Malamed, Stanley F. *Handbook of Medical Emergencies in the Dental Office.* 2nd ed. St. Louis: Mosby, 1982.

Ramani, S. Venkat. "Hysterical Seizures in the Epileptic." *Emergency Medicine* (December 15, 1982).

Robb, Preston. *Epilepsy: A Manual for Health Workers.* Washington, D.C.: U.S. Department of Health and Human Services, September 1981.

REVIEW QUESTIONS

MULTIPLE CHOICE

1. If a person experiences several epileptic seizures occuring one after the other, the person is most likely experiencing:
   a. an absence seizure
   b. status asthmaticus
   c. a partial seizure
   d. none of the above

2. In most cases epilepsy can be controlled by administering:
   a. an antidepressant
   b. an anticonvulsant
   c. an antibiotic
   d. all of the above

3. An adverse dental condition which sometimes occurs as a result of taking dilantin is:
   a. dilantin hyperplasia
   b. gingival atrophy
   c. periodontosis
   d. ANUG

4. Which of the following is not appropriate in the treatment of an epileptic seizure?
   1. loosen any tight clothing
   2. restrain the patient from making any movements
   3. remove any dental objects from the patient's mouth
   4. do not move the patient unless it is absolutely necessary
      a. 2
      b. 3, 4
      c. 1, 2, 3, 4
      d. 4

5. Which of the following may cause a person to become an epileptic?
      a. injury to the brain
      b. high fever
      c. injury during birth
      d. all the above

6. During which phase of the grand mal seizure would the tonic/clonic movements be seen?
      a. prodromal
      b. convulsive
      c. postictal
      d. none of the above

7. During what type of seizure would the patient exhibit a blank stare and twitch or blink?
      a. grand mal
      b. status epilepticus
      c. partial
      d. none of the above

8. If a person experiences an aura, it usually occurs during the _____ phase.
      a. postictal
      b. prodromal
      c. convulsive
      d. none of the above

9. Medical assistance should be summoned if:
   a. status epilepticus is suspected
   b. the patient is injured
   c. the patient stops breathing
   d. all the above

10. A petit mal seizure is most often seen in:
    a. young adults
    b. children
    c. elderly
    d. all the above

TRUE OR FALSE

F 1. All causes of epilepsy are unknown.
T 2. A patient should not be restrained during a seizure.
F 3. The most common type of epileptic seizure is a partial seizure.
T 4. The primary goal in treating an epileptic seizure is to maintain an open airway.
F 5. Anticonvulsants are not successful in treating most cases of epilepsy.
T 6. Status epilepticus causes death in 10 percent of cases.
F 7. Tonic/clonic movements are usually seen in petit mal seizures.
T 8. It is best to use fixed dental appliances, if possible, when dealing with an epileptic.
T 9. Dilantin hyperplasia occurs in some epileptics as a result of taking dilantin.
F 10. Every epileptic experiences the same type of aura.

■ CASE STUDY

Angela Harris, 32, has come to the office for the first time. When filling out the health history, she indicates that she is an epileptic. The dentist has become involved in an extensive procedure, and Angela is kept waiting in the operatory. During this time she becomes very anxious about the upcoming treatment. The dentist enters the operatory and begins treatment. The patient is very quiet and starts to twitch. She then proceeds to a full tonic/clonic seizure.

QUESTIONS

1. What could have been done to prevent the patient from experiencing the seizure?
2. How would being aware that the patient was an epileptic help during treatment of the seizure?
3. Describe the signs the patient would exhibit that would indicate this was a tonic/clonic seizure.
4. Explain the treatment that would be provided for this patient.

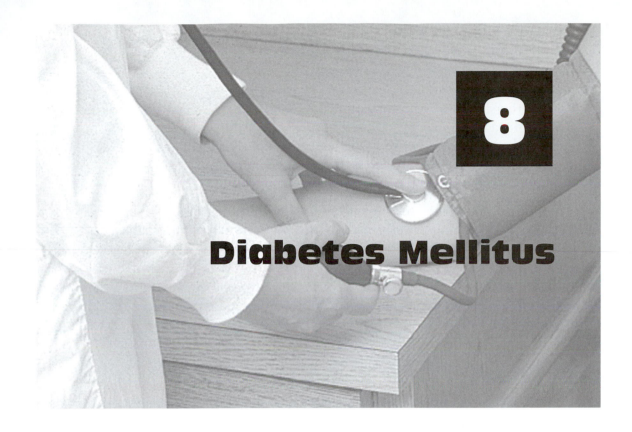

Diabetes Mellitus

KEY TERMS

Diabetic coma
Gestational diabetes
Glucagon
Glucose
Hyperglycemia
Hypoglycemia
Insulin

Insulin shock
Ketones
Macrovascular disease
Microvascular disease
Oral hypoglycemics
Pancreas
Periodontal disease

OBJECTIVES

Upon completion of this chapter the student will be able to:

- Define diabetes mellitus
- Explain the function of insulin
- Explain the difference between Type I and Type II diabetes
- Define oral hypoglycemics
- Explain two possible causes of diabetes
- Define hyperglycemia
- Explain the signs and symptoms of hyperglycemia

- Explain the treatment of hyperglycemia
- Define hypoglycemia
- Explain the signs and symptoms of hypoglycemia
- Define glucagon
- Explain the difference between diabetic coma and insulin shock
- Explain two medical problems associated with diabetes
- Describe one dental problem the diabetic may present

The term *diabetes mellitus* came from Greek and Latin sources. Diabetes is translated as "run through a siphon"; *mellitus* means "honey." Together they are said to mean "sweet water siphon." The name *diabetes mellitus* was given to this disease because medical people of ancient times observed that persons with diabetes urinated frequently and their urine tasted very sweet. Today diabetes mellitus is defined as a disease of metabolism that occurs as a result of either a deficiency or a complete lack of insulin in the body.

HISTORY

Diabetes mellitus is certainly now a new disease; it has been reported since Roman times. However, not until the early 1920s was a lack or absence of insulin discovered to be the cause of diabetes. Around 1921, insulin began to be used in the treatment of diabetes.

FUNCTIONS OF GLUCOSE AND INSULIN

Glucose is the fuel for the body that is manufactured from the food we eat. A great many of the cells of the body must have glucose to survive. Glucose is carried to all the cells by the bloodstream. However, for glucose to be able to enter the cell and provide it with the needed fuel, **insulin** (a hormone produced in the **pancreas**) must be present. In addition, the cells must also have insulin receptors. Diabetics who must take insulin suffer from a condition in which the pancreas either is not making enough insulin or not making it at all. Diabetics who do not have to take insulin have a condition in which the pancreas produces enough insulin or perhaps even too much. The problem is usually that either there are not enough insulin receptors or these receptors are defective.

It is of utmost importance that the levels of glucose in the blood be kept at appropriate levels. Although glucose is the only fuel for the brain, it is also toxic to many tissues. Too much glucose therefore has the potential to cause as many problems as too little.

This imbalance of glucose in the blood results in some complications associated with diabetes, such as **macrovascular disease**, **microvascular disease**, and neuropathy.

The imbalance also results in one of two conditions: **hypoglycemia** or **hyperglycemia**.

CLASSIFICATION

Diabetes is classified as either type I or type II.

Type I diabetes was once known as "juvenile diabetes" because it usually occurred in the young. The name was changed because the condition, although not common, has occurred in older people. A type I diabetic is insulin dependent. This means that the body does not produce adequate insulin and the person must therefore take daily insulin injections. Insulin cannot be taken orally because it is a protein and would be digested by the stomach. Type I diabetes account for about 10 percent of all of the cases of diabetes mellitus. The majority of the medical problems associated with diabetes occur in type I, usually because the patient has diabetes for such a long time.

Type II diabetes has also been known as "adult-onset diabetes." Like type I, this name was changed because this condition can also occur in the young. However, most people with type II diabetes are middle-aged and obese. Type II accounts for 90 percent of the known cases of diabetes. In most cases of type II, insulin is not required because the condition can usually be controlled with diet and, in some cases, oral hypoglycemics.

GESTATIONAL DIABETES

An additional form of diabetes is called **gestational diabetes**. This form of diabetes begins during pregnancy and ends following delivery.

Unlike type I diabetes, women with gestational diabetes have plenty of insulin. During pregnancy the placenta provides the developing fetus with nutrients and water from the mother. It also provides a variety of hormones that are vital to the pregnancy. Ironically, several of these hormones have a blocking effect on insulin. This blocking effect usually occurs approximately midway through the pregnancy. The larger the placenta becomes the more blocking of the insulin occurs. This occurs in all pregnancies and in most cases the woman is able to make additional insulin to overcome the blocking effect. However, when the pancreas makes all the insulin that it can and there still is not enough to overcome the effect of the placenta's hormones, gestational diabetes results. If the placenta's hormones from the mother's blood could be removed, the condition would end. This is what happens following delivery of the baby and therefore gestational diabetes ends when the pregnancy ends.

Any woman may develop gestational diabetes during pregnancy. However, some women are at greater risk. Some of these risk factors are obesity; a family history of diabetes; having given birth previously to a very large infant, a still birth, or a child with a birth defect; or having too much amniotic fluid. Also, women who are older than 25 are at a greater risk than younger women.

The Council on Diabetes in Pregnancy of the American Diabetes Association strongly recommends that all pregnant women be screened for gestational diabetes. The most common test is the glucose-screening test.

ORAL HYPOGLYCEMICS

Oral hypoglycemics are medications that lower blood sugar. They are not effective in treating type I diabetes, in which there is no insulin production, but they have been found to be effective in some cases of type II diabetes. Most physicians suggest that it is best to treat type II with diet control and, if medication is needed, to try insulin first. However, oral hypoglycemics are used in cases where it may be difficult or impossible for the people to give themselves insulin injections. Oral hypoglycemics are not used with pregnant patients or patients with liver or kidney problems.

CAUSES

Most causes of diabetes are not definitely known, although there are some theories. First, it is known that heredity plays a definite role in causing diabetes and that diabetes is carried by one or more genes. A person may carry this gene and yet not develop the disease, but pass it on to the next generation. Therefore, if one or both parents have diabetes, the child's chances of developing diabetes are increased.

Another theory holds that type I diabetes may have occurred as a result of a virus related to the mumps virus that damaged the cells of the pancreas, which produces insulin.

A final theory is that type II diabetes can occur as a result of pregnancy because pregnancy causes such a drastic change in the hormones of the body.

Other theories of the causes of diabetes are developing as more information concerning diabetes is discovered.

HYPERGLYCEMIA AND HYPOGLYCEMIA

The balance of glucose in the body must remain constant. If there is too much glucose, a condition known as hyperglycemia occurs. On the other hand, if there is too little sugar, a condition known as hypoglycemia occurs. Both these conditions have the potential to develop into an emergency situation.

Hyperglycemia

Hyperglycemia occurs where is too much glucose (sugar) in the blood and is usually seen when there is a deficiency or complete lack of insulin. Hyperglycemia is a slow-occurring condition. Its victim exhibits increased thirst and urination. Because of the imbalance created in the cells, there is

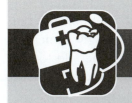

EMERGENCY BASICS

Signs of Hyperglycemia (Diabetic Coma)

Increased thirst
Increased urination
Loss of appetite
Nausea
Vomiting
Fatigue
Abdominal pains
Generalized aches

Treatment of Hyperglycemia (Diabetic Coma)

Conscious
Patient administers own insulin if available

Unconscious
Transport to medical facility

dehydration, which results in the increased thirst and ultimately increased urination. If the urine is checked there will be a large amount of sugar and **ketones**. The patient may also exhibit loss of appetite, nausea and/or vomiting, fatigue, abdominal pains, and generalized aches. If the condition is allowed to progress, the patient exhibits a heavy, labored breathing called Kussmaul breathing. The patient's breath has a fruity acetone odor as a result of the extra sugar. Without treatment, this person will lose consciousness and die. When the condition reaches this point it is called **diabetic coma**. This is also the condition present in the undiagnosed diabetic.

Diabetic coma was the most common cause of death among diabetes in the years before the discovery of insulin. Today diabetic coma should rarely occur in a known diabetic because its symptoms are identifiable for several days before the coma occurs. Also, if the diabetic is testing the urine and blood sugar on a regular basis, she will be able to determine any problems before they advance as far as diabetic coma. Diabetic coma can nevertheless kill diabetics who are not controlled.

People who suffer from hyperglycemia require insulin injections; if conscious, they should administer their own insulin. Patients suffering from diabetic coma should be taken to a medical facility. The dental staff should never attempt to administer insulin to an unconscious patient because the amount of insulin required is not known.

Hypoglycemia

Hypoglycemia, also known as **insulin shock**, occurs as a result of too little glucose in the body. Since glucose is the only source of fuel for the brain, if it goes for a long time without adequate glucose, brain-cell damage may occur.

Hypoglycemia usually has a rapid onset and may be caused by any of the following situations:

1. The diabetic may have skipped a meal or not eaten the balanced diet she requires. As a result, the insulin level is too high and the glucose level too low.

2. For some reason the patient may have experienced an unusual amount of exercise, which burned up the sugar sources within the body. Diabetics are encouraged to exercise. As a matter of fact, several famous athletes are diabetics. However, there must always be a constant balance among exercise, food, and insulin.

3. A change in routine occurs, such as when a young person goes off to college. The new patterns, schedules, and emotional stress may all cause an imbalance in the insulin and glucose levels that may result in hypoglycemia.

A person exhibiting hypoglycemia may break out in a cold sweat and appear nervous, trembling, weak, and hungry. There is usually a personality change that may include irritability, confusion, and the inability to think clearly. Often a family member or close associate of the patient may be better able to detect warning signs of hypoglycemia than the patient, since the patient may be confused. Sometimes the patient may become upset and refuse treatment as a result of confusion.

This patient requires treatment as soon as possible. Treatment for hypoglycemia includes getting some type of sugar source into the diabetic's system. If the patient is conscious, the easiest method is to give a glass of orange juice, although any good available sugar source will help. Some companies are now manufacturing a liquid sugar source that is available in a tube and is easy to administer to the patient. If the patient is unconscious, do not attempt to give anything by mouth. Instead, the person should be treated with an injection of glucagon.

Glucagon is a hormone, produced in the pancreas, that raises blood sugar. It achieves this effect by changing the sugar stored in the liver into a source of sugar that can be used by the body. As soon as hypoglycemia is diagnosed in the unconscious patient, an injection of glucagon should be given. Once the patient regains full consciousness orange juice should be administered. Glucagon is used up very quickly, and if another source of sugar is not given, the patient may relapse into hypoglycemia.

Diabetic Coma or Insulin Shock?

If you find a diabetic unconscious, it is hard to determine whether the patient is suffering from diabetic coma, insulin shock, or a related medical problem. If you have the advantage of knowing that the patient has type II diabetes and does not take insulin, you may infer that the patient is suffering from diabetic coma and should receive immediate medical attention. If you have no idea what type of diabetic you are dealing with, treat the condition as insulin shock. It is very important to get glucose into the system before the brain is damaged. A person can withstand very high levels of blood sugar much longer than the brain can survive with low levels of glucose. Therefore, if you do not know which condition the patient is suffering from, treat for insulin shock. Once this treatment is performed, if recovery does not occur, summon medical help.

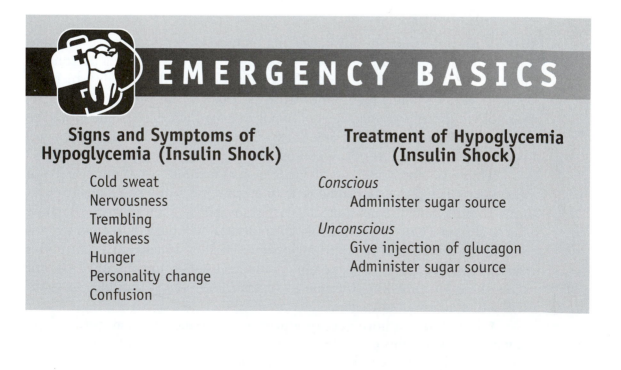

EMERGENCY BASICS

Signs and Symptoms of Hypoglycemia (Insulin Shock)

Cold sweat
Nervousness
Trembling
Weakness
Hunger
Personality change
Confusion

Treatment of Hypoglycemia (Insulin Shock)

Conscious
Administer sugar source

Unconscious
Give injection of glucagon
Administer sugar source

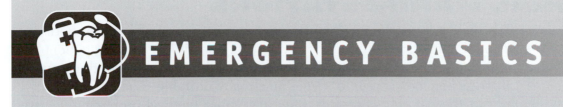

Common Medical Problems Associated with Diabetes

Macrovascular
    Myocardial infarction (see chapter 10)
    Angina pectoris (see chapter 10)
    High blood pressure
    Cerebrovascular accident (see chapter 12)
    Gangrene
    Kidney dysfunction

Microvascular
    Diabetic retinopathy

MEDICAL PROBLEMS

In addition to hypoglycemia and hyperglycemia, the diabetic also has an increased incidence of other medical problems. It is clearly known that diabetes increases the cases of *macrovascular* (large-vessel) and *microvascular* (small-vessel) abnormalities.

Large-vessel problems are indicated by:

1. inadequate blood supply to the heart muscle, resulting in conditions such as myocardial infarction or angina pectoris.
2. inadequate blood supply to the brain, resulting in various types of cerebrovascular accidents
3. inadequate blood supply to the legs, which increases the risk of infection and gangrene
4. inadequate blood supply to the kidneys, which results in kidney dysfunction or shutdown.

Small-vessel problems most often affect the small vessels of the eye. This causes a disease known as diabetic retinopathy. This problem can cause blindness in its victims.

ORAL MANIFESTATIONS

The diabetic dental patient can present some unique problems for both dentist and dental staff. First there is the strong possibility that the patient may experience diabetic coma or insulin shock while in the office—the emotional stress may be enough to trigger an already unstable situation.

If the patient is experiencing a particular medical problem associated with diabetes, such as high blood pressure or cardiovascular disease, the dental team may have to alter its treatment to avoid an emergency situation.

In addition, the diabetic may experience some specific dental problems. For example, **periodontal disease** is extremely common in diabetics. Furthermore, this periodontal disease tends to be very severe and hard to control no matter how well the patient maintains oral hygiene. There have been situations in which severe periodontal disease has caused a person's diabetes to become uncontrolled. Therefore the importance of keeping the periodontal disease to a minimum can be easily seen, and this can sometimes be achieved through good oral hygiene.

Diabetics sometimes have problems healing and are very prone to infection. This is a result of the circulatory problems associated with macrovascular and microvascular disease. The dental team, therefore, needs to be very careful and cause as little tissue trauma as possible. Furthermore, if dental surgery is performed, extra appointments should be made on a frequent basis to make sure the patient is healing properly.

When dealing with the diabetic patient, the dental team should assure the following:

1. Maintain a current, thorough medical history. It is important to realize the patient is a diabetic. It is also important to know whether she is type I or type II and if the diabetes is controlled or uncontrolled at the time of the dental appointment.
2. Consult with the patient's physician before beginning any extensive treatment. If the treatment that is to be provided will interfere with maintaining a normal routine, the patient's physician may need to make some changes in the insulin dose. There may also be some underlying medical problems that require special treatment or medication.
3. Attempt to keep the patient calm and relaxed during all phases of treatment. As previously mentioned, emotional stress or upset can trigger particular medical problems in the diabetic.
4. Avoid making appointments that would cause the patient to miss a scheduled meal. Keeping diabetes under control means keeping a good

balance among food, insulin, and exercise. Scheduling an appointment during lunch, for example, may upset the insulin balance and perhaps cause the patient to experience insulin shock.

It is very beneficial for the members of the dental team to familiarize themselves with characteristics associated with diabetes. This is extremely helpful when dealing with certain age groups of diabetics. For example, children with diabetes are sometimes concerned about experiencing new situations such as a trip to the dental office because they feel the dental staff will not understand their diabetes and therefore will not know what to do if they have any problems. It is important for each member of the team to understand diabetes not just to treat an emergency but to know how to talk and work with the patient.

In addition, adolescents may present the dental team with several emergency problems, because at this stage they tend to be very rebellious and may not be monitoring and controlling their diabetes as they should. Therefore they could experience a reaction while receiving dental treatment because their diabetes is not controlled.

SUMMARY

The real study and treatment of diabetes has only been in process for about 60 years; advancements are progressing rather rapidly and have been remarkable. New methods of diagnosing, treating, and controlling diabetes have been discovered. The space program has resulted in several advancements in the treatment of diabetes. Hopefully, in the near future, advancements will be made and the dental team will no longer have to deal with problems such as diabetic coma or insulin shock.

REFERENCES

Anderson, Carol E. "Explaining the Genetic Risks for Siblings and Offspring." *Consultant* (October 1982).

Biermann, June, and Barbara Toohey. *The Diabetic's Book*. Tarcher, 1981.

Bovington, Mary M., Martha Enzenauer Spies, and Patrick J. Troy. "Management of the Patient with Diabetes Mellitus During Surgery or Illness." *Nursing Clinics of North America 18* (December 1983).

Duncan, Theodore G. *The Diabetes Fact Book*. New York: Scribner, 1982.

Feingold, Kenneth R. "How Emotions Affect Blood Glucose Levels." *Consultant* (November 1982).

Guthrie, Diane W., and Richard A. Guthrie. "The Disease Process of Diabetes Mellitus: Definition, Characteristics, Trends, and Developments." *Nursing Clinics of North America 18* (December 1983).

Hoette, Sharon J. "The Adolescent with Diabetes Mellitus." *Nursing Clinics of North America 18* (December 1983).

Krauser, Kathleen L., and Paul B. Madden. "The Child with Diabetes Mellitus." *Nursing Clinics of North America 18* (December 1983).

Moorman, Nicky Harmon. "Acute Complications of Hyperglycemia and Hypoglycemia." *Nursing Clinics of North America 18* (December 1983).

Muggeo, M., (1998) "Accelerated complications in Type II diabetes mellitus; the need for greater awareness and earlier detection." *Diabetic Medicine*.

Passa, P., (1998) "Reducing the cardiovascular consequences of diabetes mellitus." *Diabetic Medicine*.

Price, Martha J. "Insulin and Oral Hypoglycemia Agents." *Nursing Clinics of North America 18* (December 1983).

Rose, Louise T., Barry H. Hendler, and James T. Amsterdam. "Orofacial Pain and Manifestations of Systemic Disease." *Consultant* (November 1982).

Spies, Martha Enzenauer. "Vascular Complications Associated with Diabetes Mellitus." *Nursing Clinics of North America 18* (December 1983).

Stock-Barkman, Patricia. "Confusing Concepts: Is It Diabetic Shock or Diabetic Coma?" *Nursing 13* (June 1983)

Trevisan, R., Vedovato, M., & Tiengo, A., (1998) "The epidemiology of diabetes mellitus." *Nephrology Dialysis Transplantation 13*, 2–5.

Wolinsky, Harvey. "Diabetes Mellitus and Cardiovascular Complications." *Consultant* (July 1981).

Zoeller, Gilbert N., and Barney Kadis. "The Diabetic Dental Patient." *General Dentistry* (January-February 1981).

REVIEW QUESTIONS

MULTIPLE CHOICE

1. Type I diabetes is most often treated with daily injections of:
   a. glucagon
   b. insulin
   c. oral hypoglycemics
   d. glucose

2. Type II diabetes may sometimes be treated with:
   a. oral hypoglycemics
   b. glucagon
   c. glucose
   d. none of the above

3. Which of the following are signs or symptoms of hyperglycemia?
   1. increased thirst
   2. Kussmaul breathing
   3. confusion
   4. increased urination
      a. 1, 2, 3, 4
      b. 1, 2, 3
      c. 1, 2, 4
      d. 2, 3, 4

4. Diabetic coma is treated with:
   a. glucagon
   b. glucose
   c. insulin
   d. none of the above

5. Which of the following are not signs or symptoms of insulin shock?
   1. rapid onset
   2. cold sweat
   3. confusion
   4. increased thirst
      a. 1, 2
      b. 3, 4
      c. 1
      d. 4

6. The unconscious patient suffering from insulin shock should be treated by:
   a. giving orange juice
   b. administering insulin injection
   c. administering oral hypoglycemics
   d. administering glucagon injection

7. An example of a microvascular disease is:
   a. angina pectoris
   b. diabetic retinopathy
   c. kidney dysfunction
   d. cerebrovascular accident

8. The only fuel for the brain is:
   a. glucose
   b. insulin
   c. glucagon
   d. none of the above

9. The correct treatment for the conscious patient suffering from insulin shock is to:
   a. administer a sugar source such as orange juice
   b. administer insulin
   c. administer a glucagon injection
   d. none of the above

10. The diabetic dental patient may be more prone to:
    a. decay
    (b.) periodontal disease
    c. malocclusion
    d. all the above

TRUE OR FALSE

T 1. Insulin may not be taken orally because it is digested by the stomach.
F 2. Most medical problems are associated with type II diabetes.
T 3. Diabetic coma was the leading cause of death among diabetics before the discovery of insulin.
F 4. Type II diabetes was once called juvenile diabetes.
F 5. Diabetes is a disease that originated in the early 1900s.
T 6. Type II diabetes accounts for 90 percent of the diagnosed cases of diabetes.
F 7. Type I diabetes can usually be controlled with diet.
T 8. Heredity plays an important part in the cause of diabetes.
T 9. Insulin is produced in the body by the pancreas.
F 10. Hypoglycemia results when there is too much sugar in the bloodstream.

■ CASE STUDY

Mollie Norris, a 35-year-old diabetic, is scheduled for an amalgam. Before her appointment, the dental assistant checks her health history and finds that she is a type I diabetic taking daily injections of insulin. Mollie rushes into the office slightly late for her appointment. She reports that she was in such a hurry she did not get a chance to eat lunch. As the appointment begins, Mollie breaks out in a cold sweat and appears very nervous. When the dentist questions her, she seems confused.

QUESTIONS

1. What condition is Mollie most likely suffering from?
2. What should be done to treat this condition?
3. How might this situation have been avoided?

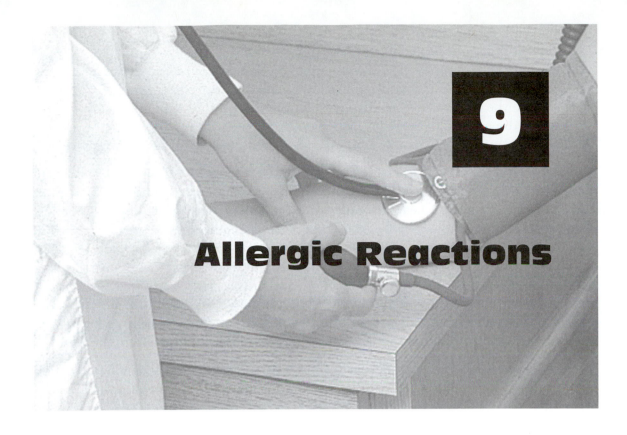

Allergic Reactions

KEY TERMS

Anaphylaxis
Angioedema
Antibody
Antigen
Cardiac arrhythmias
Contact dermatitis

Histamine
Immune system
Immunoglobulin system
Latex allergy
Urticaria

OBJECTIVES

Upon completion of this chapter the student will be able to:

- Describe the functions of the immunoglobulin system
- Explain what must take place for an allergic reaction to occur
- Explain the special importance of a thorough medical history when dealing with an allergic patient
- Explain the signs, symptoms, and treatment for allergic skin reactions
- Define an anaphylactic reaction
- Describe the signs and symptoms associated with an anaphylactic reaction
- Explain the treatment for an anaphylactic reaction with allergic symptoms

- Explain the treatment for an anaphylactic reaction without allergic symptoms
- Describe the role of epinephrine in treating allergic reactions
- Describe the steps to follow when a patient is allergic to dental anesthesia
- Explain the signs and symptoms associated with latex allergy
- Describe the protocol to follow when a staff member or patient is allergic to latex

Mary Henderson has an appointment with the dentist to have a class I amalgam placed in tooth number 20. Upon examining her medical history, the auxiliary notes that Mary is in excellent health except for listing allergies to dust, penicillin, sulfur drugs, insect stings, and seafood. The dentist administers the anesthesia, and within 30 seconds the patient begins to exhibit problems. She complains that it feels as if her throat is closing; she is nauseated, itches all over, and is becoming very anxious. The dentist diagnoses acute anaphylactic reaction. The auxiliary immediately transmits the epinephrine-loaded syringe to the dentist. This is administered by the dentist, and the patient begins to recover. This patient was experiencing a severe anaphylactic reaction to the anesthesia. Without proper treatment, she would have died within minutes.

A vast majority of the population is allergic to one thing or another. The reaction to this allergy may range from a slight rash and runny nose to a fatal anaphylactoid reaction.

To understand an allergic reaction, it is important to understand the functions and makeup of the body's **immune system**.

ANTIBODIES

An **antibody**, which is produced by the lymphoid tissues, is an essential part of the body's immune system. Antibodies are produced when a virus, bacteria, or some other foreign substance enters the body. A particular type of antibody is produced for each foreign substance, which is called an allergen or **antigen**. So far, five different classifications of antibodies have been discovered. Together they make up the **immunoglobulin system** (Emergency Basics).

Immunoglobulin A (IgA) is the most prevalent antibody. It is found in all the secretions of the body and helps protect the body from dangerous microorganisms.

Immunoglobulin D (IgD) is found in serum tissue. The function of the IgD antibody has not been determined.

Immunoglobulin E (IgE) is a very important antibody found in the lungs, skin, and cells of mucous membrane. IgE is responsible for reacting

EMERGENCY BASICS

Immunoglobulin System

IgA fights microorganisms
IgD function unknown
IgE initiates type I reactions
IgG provides unborn with immunity
IgM first defense against microorganisms

with certain antigens and causing type I reactions, which are anaphylactic reactions.

Immunoglobulin G (IgG) also helps protect the body from invading microorganisms. It is best known for crossing the placenta and providing the unborn with immunity.

Immunoglobulin M (IgM) is the first antibody the body produces when an antigen enters.

ANTIGEN

An *antigen*, sometimes called an *allergen*, is a substance that enters the body and can produce a hypersensitive reaction but is not necessarily intrinsically harmful. Most people develop a natural or acquired immunity to allergens, but in people who suffer from allergies, the body is overly sensitive to the antigen. When an allergic reaction occurs, the body's immune system is not protecting itself against the allergen.

ALLERGIC REACTION

When an antigen enters a body, the body's defense mechanism goes into play. Basic defense mechanisms such as the skin, the lining of the nasal passages, and the like attempt to block the antigen from entering the system. If this does not work and the antigen enters the system, the immunoglobulin system goes into action. In most cases the antigen is destroyed. If for some reason the antigen is not destroyed, certain chemicals may be released that may result in various degrees of allergic reactions.

Prerequisites for Reactions

A person does not experience an allergic reaction during the first exposure to the antigen. For example, a person who is going to be allergic to penicillin does not experience any reaction the first time the drug is given. This first dose is known as the sensitizing dose. After this dose, the body produces the IgE antibody, which reacts only to this particular antigen. For a period after exposure, the IgE antibody continues to be produced while the antigen decreases. After a certain time, only the specific IgE antibody is circulating in the body. At this point no allergic reaction occurs.

When the person is exposed to this same allergen, or one chemically similar, an allergic reaction does occur. This results as the body recognizes the antigen and chemical elements that cause the reaction are released. The main chemical is **histamine**. Histamine is found in all cells but is only released in allergic reactions. It has the ability to cause dilation of the capillaries, increased secretion of the gastric juices, decreased blood pressure, and constriction of some of the smooth muscles.

The type of allergic reaction that results depends mainly on the type and amount of allergen involved.

IMPORTANCE OF MEDICAL HISTORY

The medical history is never more important than when dealing with the allergy-prone patient.

It has been determined that a person with a history of allergies to several substances (such as pollen, eggs, seafood, and penicillin) is very likely to experience an allergic reaction to some item or drug used in the dental office. Evidently this person's body responses are highly sensitized, and the patient requires special attention during the procedures.

In addition, the medical history is important in telling the dental staff what substances have actually caused the patient to experience an allergic reaction. For example, if a patient reports experience in the past of an allergic reaction to xylocaine, the dental team would not use this particular drug during the procedure.

TYPES OF REACTION

Allergic reactions vary in type and severity. The reaction may occur almost immediately because of the humoral system or may be delayed for several days as a result of the cell-mediated system. The reaction may be localized to one area, such as a skin reaction, or may be generalized, involving the whole body, as in an anaphylactoid reaction.

In some instances it is possible to predetermine the severity of a reaction. It is known that the time that elapses between exposure to the allergen and the onset of the allergic reaction determines to a great extent the severity of the reaction. If some reaction is noticed within a few minutes of exposure, the reaction may be much more severe than when the reaction is seen several hours to a few days after the exposure.

Skin Reactions

There is a wide variety of skin disorders, ranging from mild to very severe. Skin reactions may also be the first stage of anaphylactoid reactions. So, no matter how mild it seems, the progression should always be watched carefully.

Contact Dermatitis

Contact dermatitis is an allergic skin reaction that occurs as a result of cutaneous exposure to a particular allergen and may occur in the oral mucosa as well as in the skin. The allergen that may cause this type of reaction can include such things as poison ivy, toothpaste, mouthwash, lipstick or other cosmetics, impression materials, metal alloys, and stainless steel wire, to name only a few.

Contact dermatitis is usually an acute problem, but if the allergen is not removed and exposure continues, the condition becomes chronic and in some cases disabling.

The first signs of contact dermatitis include erythema (redness), edema (swelling), and vesicle (blister) formation. In some intense cases these vesicles may rupture and result in an open, oozing wound. The main symptom is intense itching. This symptom, as well as the condition, is usually localized to the one area where the antigen contacted the surface, although in a few cases it may spread.

In most cases the first step of treatment is to remove the contactants. A physician may further administer corticosteroids and antihistamines.

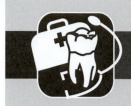

EMERGENCY BASICS

Contact Dermatitis

Signs and Symptoms
    itching
    erythema
    edema
    vesicle formation

Treatment
    remove contactants
    antihistamine
    corticosteroids

Urticaria

Urticaria is a skin condition most of the general public calls hives. It may be caused by any substance that is either ingested or placed on the skin surface. This condition consists of circumscribed raised areas of erythema and edema and, as with any allergic reaction, it may be mild or severe.

As with contact dermatitis, the main course of treatment is to remove the substance. For example, if the urticaria was caused by some substance

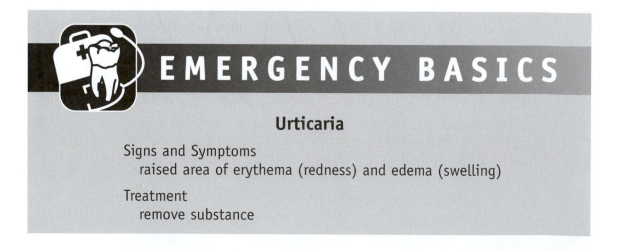

EMERGENCY BASICS

Urticaria

Signs and Symptoms
    raised area of erythema (redness) and edema (swelling)

Treatment
    remove substance

that the patient ingested, the course of treatment would be to stop the ingestion of the substance.

ANGIOEDEMA

In its beginning stages, **angioedema**—also called angioneurotic edema—is sometimes mistaken for urticaria, and, basically, angioedema is a giant form of urticaria. It is characterized by localized swelling of either the submucosa or subcutaneous tissues. The lesions associated with angioedema have certain characteristics: usually the lesions are single but in some cases they may be multiple; they are very large and do not have defined raised borders like urticaria; and there is no pain and usually no associated itching.

The tissues of the genitals, face, and hands are the areas usually affected by angioedema. Angioedema is usually caused by an allergic reaction to drugs, food, infection, and so on.

As with most skin reactions, angioedema occurs when an antigen enters the body, histamine is released, capillaries dilate, and fluid enters the area.

It is commonly seen in people with a history of various allergies but may also be found in those with no allergy history.

Treatment consists of removing the cause and administering an antihistamine. In most cases this reverses the situation without giving it a chance to

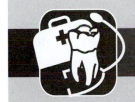

EMERGENCY BASICS

Angioedema

Signs and Symptoms
- localized swelling of submucosa
- localized swelling of subcutaneous tissue
- usually single lesions
- no pain
- no itching

Treatment
- remove the cause
- administer antihistamine

cause major problems. However, if this occurs in the dental office, the team should watch the patient carefully for a time to make sure the swelling does not increase in a certain area where it may have the potential to inhibit respiration.

Note that in most mild cases of allergic skin reactions, the dentist may choose not to treat the patient in the dental office but rather refer the patient to a physician or allergist. This action may prove satisfactory, but the dental team should observe the patient and always provide follow-up treatment either in the office or by referral.

Most skin reactions do not create emergency situations in themselves. The big danger is that skin reactions may either advance and create an emergency or be the beginning of a true emergency situation such as anaphylactic shock.

RESPIRATORY ALLERGIC REACTION

Allergic reactions that may affect only the respiratory system also occur. The most common type of respiratory reaction is asthma, covered in detail in chapter 5.

ANAPHYLACTIC REACTION

An anaphylactic reaction is a severe allergic reaction that occurs in previously sensitized patients. It develops almost immediately after the patient ingests, inhales, or is injected with an antigen or is stung by an insect. **Anaphylaxis** is the most severe allergic reaction and often proves fatal regardless of the treatment administered.

Physiology

As with other allergic reactions, anaphylaxis occurs only in those who have been previously exposed to the allergen. The patient is exposed to the allergen, an incubation period takes place, and antibodies form. When the patient is exposed to the same allergen, the anaphylactic reaction occurs. This is sometimes called the exciting or shock dose, which is how the name anaphylactic shock came into existence.

Severity

Symptoms associated with anaphlaxis can vary in a wide range of severity that depends on the amount of acquired sensitivity, the amount of antigen that entered the body, and the method in which the antigen entered the body. Furthermore, the time that elapses between the exposure to the antigen and the onset of symptoms usually indicates how serious the reaction will be. For example, reactions that occur within the first 30 minutes after contact with the antigen are usually the most severe. Reactions that occur after 30 minutes are less likely to be fatal.

Symptoms

Signs and symptoms associated with anaphylaxis vary in both type and severity. These may be seen in the skin, gastrointestinal, respiratory, or circulatory systems.

Signs or symptoms associated with the skin may include generalized pruritus, urticaria, or angioedema. Normally these conditions are not too dangerous, but they do have the potential to become life-threatening if they are located in some specific areas. For example, angioedema located around the mouth or throat could cause death from airway obstruction. Gastrointestinal signs and symptoms may include varying degrees of nausea, vomiting, and diarrhea.

Respiratory signs and symptoms may include varying degrees of airway obstruction. This most often occurs as a result of laryngeal edema, a swelling of the larynx that occurs as a result of an allergic reaction. The swelling may be great enough to cause partial or even complete obstruction of the airway. It is the most common cause of death in anaphylactic reactions.

Circulatory signs and symptoms may include hypotension, shock, **cardiac arrhythmias**, and even complete circulatory collapse.

All the signs and symptoms associated with an anaphylactic reaction vary in their severity as well as in the way they present themselves. Diagnosis can nevertheless be relatively easy if the signs and symptoms occur right after the exposure.

For example, almost immediately after exposure the patient feels faint and weak, begins sweating, and becomes anxious and restless. The patient then develops a severe itching sensation as a result of allergic skin reactions. The condition then proceeds through the gastrointestinal, respiratory, and circulatory stages. If this cycle is not stopped, the end result will be death.

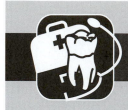

EMERGENCY BASICS

Anaphylaxis

Signs and symptoms
    Skin
        generalized pruritus *itching*
        urticaria
        angioedema
    Gastrointestinal
        nausea
        vomiting
        diarrhea
    Respiratory
        laryngeal edema
    Circulatory
        hypotension
        shock
        cardiac arrhythmias
        complete circulatory collapse
    Plus:
        sweating
        anxious feeling
        nervousness

One special problem associated with anaphylactic shock is that in some cases the reaction can be so severe that all the signs and symptoms occur at once. In these situations diagnosis may be more difficult and death may occur in spite of any treatment.

Treatment

At the very first sign of an anaphylactic reaction, place the patient in a supine position and administer oxygen. The receptionist should summon medical assistance. In the meantime, the auxiliary should get the emergency kit and

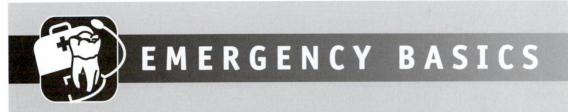

EMERGENCY BASICS

Treatment with Obvious Signs and Symptoms

1. summon medical assistance
2. place the patient in a supine position
3. administer oxygen
4. administer epinephrine
5. administer antihistamine as needed
6. perform cricothyrotomy if needed
7. initiate CPR if needed

EMERGENCY BASICS

Treatment of an Anaphylactic Reaction Without Signs or Symptoms

1. summon medical assistance
2. do not administer epinephrine
3. place patient in Trendelenburg position
4. provide basic life support as needed
5. initiate CPR if needed
6. perform cricothyrotomy if needed

prepare an epinephrine injection; the dentist should administer the epinephrine immediately. Remember that a subsequent injection of epinephrine may be required. If more than one injection of epinephrine is needed, the dentist may given an injection of antihistamine during the acute phase. During this entire time, attention must be paid to the patient's airway, since laryngeal edema may occur to block the airway. However, once the epinephrine is administered, the patient's condition should improve. If laryngeal edema occurs and complete airway obstruction results, aid the dentist in performing a cricothyrotomy. If there is a complete loss of blood pressure and/or pulse, the dentist and auxiliary should begin CPR until medical assistance arrives.

The treatment is specific for an anaphylactic reaction that demonstrates the signs and symptoms mentioned earlier. The problem unique to the anaphylactic reaction is that sometimes the reaction can be so severe that the signs and symptoms occur so quickly they all seem to happen at once. In this situation the patient may become unconscious almost immediately. In this case it is hard to determine that this condition was caused by an allergic reaction. If there are no definitive signs of an allergic reaction, the dentist should not administer epinephrine. Instead the patient should be placed in the Trendelenburg position, basic life support provided as needed with extra attention paid to maintaining the airway, and medical assistance summoned. If the condition worsens, CPR or cricothyrotomy may become necessary.

EPINEPHRINE

In the treatment of severe allergic reactions, epinephrine is the drug of choice. Epinephrine is a vasopressor, has antihistaminic action, and is a bronchodilator. Its effect is extremely rapid in onset. This characteristic in particular makes it especially useful in the treatment of anaphylactic reactions when time is crucial.

Although epinephrine is extremely beneficial in the treatment of allergic reactions, it should never be administered unless you are sure the patient is suffering from an allergic reaction. Some conditions, such as cerebral vascular accident, may at first be mistaken for an allergic reaction, since the patient may lose consciousness; administering epinephrine, which increases blood pressure, could possibly cause extreme harm.

ALLERGY TO ANESTHESIA

Once aspect of allergic reactions unique to dentistry is an allergic reaction to dental anesthetic solutions.

If a dental patient reports on the medical history an allergy to dental anesthesia, the dentist should explore a little further. Many patients are denied treatment with anesthesia because they have been told they were allergic to anesthesia when their reaction was actually a result of some other problem or was of some type other than allergic. It has been estimated that fewer than 1 percent of all bad reactions to anesthesia are actually allergic.

However, there are cases in which the patient is actually allergic to the anesthesia and will indeed experience an allergic reaction. The majority of reactions are characterized by inflammation, papules, edema, and pruritus. Nevertheless, the response can be severe enough to cause an anaphylactic reaction. These should be treated according to the section on treatment. Luckily, patients who are allergic to one type of anesthesia can sometimes be given anesthesia from another chemical group to which they are not allergic.

LATEX ALLERGIES

Allergy to natural rubber latex is now being recognized as an increasing serious medical problem that affects not only health workers, but also the general population. The incidence of **latex allergies** has increased dramatically since the 1980s.

Allergic reactions to latex can range from minor skin irritations to fatal anaphylactic reactions. Because the minor skin reactions mimic so many common situations they are often overlooked by the individual or even misdiagnosed by physicians.

Individuals at Risk for Latex Allergies

Both individuals with a genetic history of allergies and individuals with a high exposure to latex products are at an increased risk for latex hypersensitivity. In these instances the risk tends to increase with greater exposure.

Some studies have stated that 8% to 12% of health care workers with regular exposure to latex are sensitized, as compared to 1% to 6% of the general public. This percentage, especially with regard to health care workers, continues to increase.

Additional risk factors may also include a history of surgery, especially during childhood, spina bifida, disorders requiring repeated urinary catheterization, and certain food allergies including bananas, avocados, chestnuts, and kiwi.

Although a high incidence occurs in health care workers, a dental office must also prepare to see patients with this same allergy.

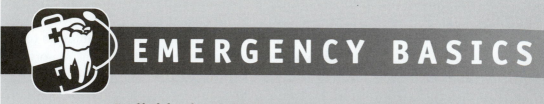

Individuals at high risk for latex allergies

- Health care workers
- Individuals with a genetic history of allergies
- Individuals with a history of surgery at a young age
- Spina bifida patients
- Individuals with disorders requiring repeated urinary catheterization
- Individuals with food allergies including bananas, avocadoes, chestnuts, and kiwi

Signs and Symptoms of Latex Allergy

Three different types of reactions may be seen in individuals who are allergic to latex. The most common is contact dermatitis. This may result in dry, itchy, irritated areas of the skin, usually the hands. This results from exposure to latex products. The second type of reaction is a delayed contact reaction. This type of reaction is very similar to poison ivy reactions. It typically occurs 48 to 72 hours after exposure and may include a red, itchy rash or possibly blisters. This type of reaction has been found to be the most common reaction.

The third type of reaction is the immediate allergic reaction. The signs of this reaction usually occur 2 to 3 minutes after contact with the latex. In this situation the individual may experience itching at the area of contact followed by welts or rash. These signs may disappear within 30 minutes. Additional immediate reactions may occur in individuals with sensitivity to airborne allergens associated with latex. This is commonly associated with powder used with latex gloves. This powder can be released as a result of putting on or removing gloves as well as by removing gloves from the glove box. The latex particles attach themselves to the powder and become airborne. As a result, sensitized individuals may experience coughing, wheezing, shortness of breath, and respiratory distress. The severity of the reaction depends on the sensitivity of the individual. In extreme cases, where sensitivity is extremely high, an anaphylactic reaction may occur.

EMERGENCY BASICS

Reactions to Latex Allergies

- Contact dermatitis
- Delayed contact reaction
- Immediate allergic reaction

Treatment

Currently there is no cure for latex allergy. Prevention and avoidance of exposure to latex and treatment of symptoms are the main treatment options.

Should one of the three types of reactions previously stated occur in a staff member or a patient, the treatment should be provided as discussed in the previous sections of this chapter.

Prevention

Individuals must be tested by a physician to determine that they have a true allergy to latex. In individuals in which this has been diagnosed, steps should be taken to prevent exposure to latex.

In order to minimize exposure to latex, sensitized dental staff members should:

- Use non-latex gloves and products
- Learn to recognize the signs and symptoms of latex allergy
- Avoid areas where you might inhale the powder from latex gloves worn by others
- Inform employer and staff of your allergy
- Wear a medical alert bracelet

When treating a patient who indicates a diagnosed allergy to latex, the following steps should be implemented:

- When possible schedule this person as the first patient of the day
- No latex products should be in the treatment room

- The treatment room should be prepared/set-up with non-latex gloves
- Instruments should be handled with non-latex gloves
- Wear non-latex gloves during treatment
- Use latex-free materials and instruments

Information on latex allergies continues to develop. New products that are latex-free are entering the market on a daily basis. All dental professionals should continue to seek education on this topic and continue to make changes as more information becomes available.

SUMMARY

Allergic reactions in the dental office can be fatal. The amount of treatment the auxiliary is allowed to perform, although not lacking in importance, is somewhat limited. Since the main method of treatment in severe reactions is an injection of epinephrine, the treatment must be performed by the dentist. It is nevertheless very important for the auxiliary to understand what takes place during a reaction and assist the dentist by having all drugs prepared. Remember, in an anaphylactic reaction, death can occur quickly if correct treatment is not provided. The auxiliary should also help the dentist administer CPR if this becomes necessary.

A smooth working team will make the treatment run smoothly, which will benefit everyone involved.

REFERENCES

Brodoff, Ami S. "Keeping Current on Allergy Treatment." *Patient Care* (February 15, 1984).

Buckley, Rebecca H., and Kenneth P. Matthews. "Common Allergic Skin Disorders." *Journal of the American Medical Association 248* (November 26, 1982).

Cohen, Steven H., and Jordan N. Fink. "The Allergic Patient: Office Evaluation." *Hospital Medicine* (February 1983).

Donlon, William C. "Immunology in Dentistry." *Journal of the American Dental Association 100* (February 1980).

Fisher, Alexander A. "Allergic Reactions of Topical Medications." *Consultant* (June 1979).

Hallock, James A. "Managing Anaphylaxis in Children." *Consultant* (July 1980).

Hunt, L.W., et al. "A medical-center-wide, multidisciplinary approach to the problem of natural rubber latex allergy." *Journal of Occupational and Environmental Medicine* 38(8):765-770.

Johnson, William T., and Time DeStigter. "Hypersensitivity to Procaine, Tetracaine, Mepivacaine, and Methylparaben: Report of a Case." *Journal of the American Dental Association 106* (January 1983).

Katelaris, C.H., Widmer, R.P., Lazarus, R.M. "Prevalence of latex allergy in dental schools." *The Medical Journal of Australia*, 1998, 164:711-714.

Kramer, Howard S., and Von A. Mitton. "Complications of Local Anesthesia." *Dental Clinics of North America 17* (July 1973).

Matthews, Kenneth P. "Respiratory Atopic Disease." *Journal of the American Medical Association 248* (November 26, 1982).

McCarthy, Frank M. *Medical Emergencies in Dentistry*. Philadelphia: Saunders, 1982.

O'Hollaren, M.T., (1998) "Update in allergy and immunology." *Annals of Internal Medicine, 129* 1036–1043.

Patterson, Roy, and Martin Valentine. "Anaphylaxis and Related Allergic Emergencies Including Reactions Due to Insect Stings." *Journal of the American Medical Association 248* (November 26, 1982).

Seskin, Leonard. "Anaphylaxis Due to Local Anesthesia Hypersensitivity: Report of a Case." *Journal of the American Dental Association 96* (May 1978).

Shepard, Felix E., Peter C. Moon, George C. Grant, and Lincoln D. Fretwell. "Allergic Contact Stomatitis from a Gold Alloy-Fixed Partial Denture." *Journal of the American Dental Association 106* (February 1983).

REVIEW QUESTIONS

MULTIPLE CHOICE

1. The immunoglobulin responsible for causing type I allergic reactions is:
   a. IgA
   b. IgE
   c. IgG
   d. IgM

2. The foreign substance that enters the body and causes an allergic reactions is a/an:
   a. antibody
   b. lymph cell
   c. immunoglob
   (d.) antigen

3. An allergic skin reaction that occurs as a result of direct exposure of the skin to a particular allergen is:
   (a.) contact dermatitis
   b. angioedema
   c. urticaria
   d. laryngeal edema

4. An allergic skin reaction that is also known as hives is:
   a. contact dermatitis
   b. angioedema
   (c.) urticaria
   d. laryngeal edema

5. The treatment for angioedema consists of:
   a. removing the cause
   b. administering an antibiotic
   c. administering an antihistamine
   (d.) a and c

6. The most common type of allergic respiratory reaction is:
   a. emphysema
   b. bronchitis
   c. tuberculosis
   (d.) none of the above

7. The most important part of treating an anaphylactic reaction consists of administering:
   a. oxygen
   b. antihistamine
   c. corticosteroid
   (d.) epinephrine

8. The most common cause of death associated with an anaphylactic reaction is:
   a. hypotension
   b. laryngeal edema
   c. cardiovascular collapse
   d. none of the above

9. Which of the following is a function of histamine?
   a. dilation of the capillaries
   b. secretion of gastric juices
   c. decreased blood pressure
   d. all the above

10. Which of the following are areas of the body most often affected by angioedema?
    1. torso
    2. hands
    3. face
    4. genitals
       a. 1, 2, 3, 4
       b. 1, 2, 4
       c. 2, 3, 4
       d. 2, 3

TRUE OR FALSE

T 1. A patient who is allergic to one type of dental anesthesia may be able to tolerate another type.

F 2. A patient usually experiences an allergic reaction on first exposure to the harmful antigen.

T 3. The time that elapses between exposure to an antigen and the onset of symptoms helps in determining the severity of the upcoming reaction.

T 4. The patient with a history of allergies to several things is a likely candidate for an allergic reaction in the dental office.

F 5. The main symptom of contact dermatitis is swelling.

T 6. It is not uncommon for a person to die from a severe anaphylactic reaction even if proper treatment is provided.

T 7. Signs and symptoms associated with an anaphylactic reaction may be seen in the skin, gastrointestinal, respiratory, or circulatory system.

F 8. The signs and symptoms of an anaphylactic reaction never occur so rapidly that they cannot be distinguished.

T 9. A dentist who is not sure the patient is suffering from an anaphylactic reaction should not administer epinephrine.

T 10. Patients who state they once experienced an allergic reaction to dental anesthesia should be checked out by an allergist.

■ CASE STUDY

Jake Matthews, an 18-year-old in good general health, has an appointment with the dentist for the extraction of the upper right third molar. Upon checking the health history, the auxiliary notes that there are no problems or allergies noted. The dentist enters the operatory and administers the injection of anesthesia. In less than a minute the patient loses consciousness. There are no signs or symptoms of allergy.

QUESTIONS

1. What should be the first step in treating this patient? *call 911, then Trendelenburg position*
2. Should epinephrine be administered? *No*
3. Should medical help be summoned? *Yes*

Angina Pectoris and Myocardial Infarction

10

KEY TERMS

Amyl nitrite
Aorta
Arteriosclerosis
Atherosclerosis
Atria
Atrioventricular valves
Endocardium
Epicardium
Epigastrium

Myocardium
Nitroglycerin
Orthostatic hypotension
Pericardium
Pulmonary artery
Semilunar valves
Vasodilator
Ventricles

OBJECTIVES

Upon completion of this chapter the student will be able to:

- Name the major parts of the heart
- Explain how atherosclerosis affects the coronary arteries

- Define angina pectoris
- Explain the difference between stable and unstable angina. List three precipitating factors of angina
- Describe the signs and symptoms of angina
- Explain how the dentist may diagnose angina
- Describe the treatment for angina
- List two side effects of nitroglycerin
- Define myocardial infarction
- Describe the signs and symptoms of myocardial infarction
- Describe the treatment for myocardial infarction
- Describe the two differences between angina and myocardial infarction
- Explain how stress is a precipitating factor of angina
- Explain what the dental team can do to prevent angina or myocardial infarction from occurring in the dental office

Today the mere mention of heart attack, heart disease, or cardiovascular disease strikes fear into most people. This fear is not entirely unjustified, since cardiovascular disease is the major cause of death in the United States today. Heart disease may present itself in several ways, but this chapter is limited to two types of heart disease that may present emergency situations in the dental office: angina pectoris and acute myocardial infarction.

ANATOMY OF THE HEART

To understand how certain diseases or conditions affect the heart, it is important to understand some of the basic anatomy of the heart.

Several structures combine to make up the four-chambered, hollow, muscular organ known as the heart (Figure 10-1). First, the **pericardium** is the wall, or sac, that encloses the heart. This wall is made up of three layers: the external layer, called the **epicardium**; the middle layer, called the **myocardium**; and the inner layer, called the **endocardium**. Each layer has special characteristics or responsibilities. First, coronary vessels must pass through the epicardium before entering the myocardium. Second, the myocardium consists of muscle fibers that give the heart the ability to contract. Third, the endocardium lines the cavities of the heart, covers the valves, and, to some extent, lines the large blood vessels.

The heart consists of four chambers. The upper chambers are called the **atria** and are separated into right and left sides by the interatrial septum. The lower chambers are called the **ventricles** and are divided into right and left sides by the interventricular septum.

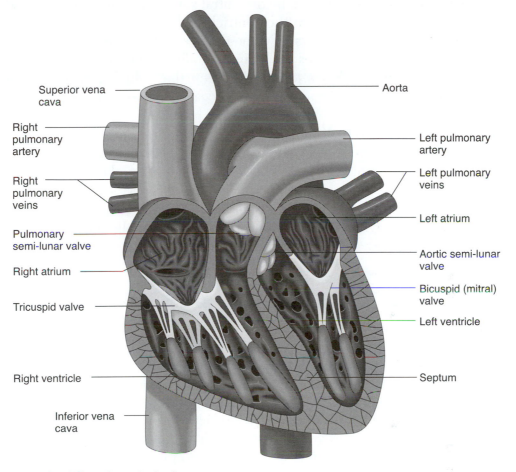

Superior vena
cava

Right
pulmonary
artery

Right
pulmonary
veins

Pulmonary
semi-lunar valve

Right atrium

Tricuspid valve

Right ventricle

Inferior vena
cava

Aorta

Left pulmonary
artery

Left pulmonary
veins

Left atrium

Aortic semi-lunar
valve

Bicuspid (mitral)
valve

Left ventricle

Septum

Figure 10-1 Blood flow through the heart

 The right atrium receives blood from all tissues except the lungs. This blood is then pumped to the right ventricle, from which the **pulmonary artery** exits and carries blood to the lungs. The left atrium receives oxygenated blood from the lungs by way of the pulmonary veins. The left ventricle is connected to the **aorta**, which pumps blood to all parts of the body except the lungs.

 Contained within the heart's chambers are two kinds of valves: the **atrioventricular valves**, which consist of the tricuspid and mitral valves, and the **semilunar valves**, which consist of the pulmonary and aortic valves. The atrioventricular valves separate the atria from the ventricles. The right atrium and ventricle are separated by the tricuspid valve, and the left atrium and ventricle are separated by the mitral valve. The valves allow blood to be pumped from the atria to the ventricles when the atria contract and then prevent blood from reversing when the ventricles contract.

The semilunar valves work similarly, although their location is different. The pulmonary valve is located between the right ventricle and the pulmonary artery, and the aortic valve is located between the left ventricle and the aorta.

The heart is best known as the organ that provides blood to the rest of the body, but, to survive, the heart muscle itself must receive an adequate supply of oxygenated blood. The myocardium is supplied with blood by the first branches of the aorta, the right and left coronary arteries. The left coronary artery branches to supply blood to the left and right ventricles and left atrium. The right coronary artery branches and supplies blood to the left and right ventricles and the right atrium.

CORONARY ARTERY DISEASE

Both physical and emotional stress can cause the heart to work harder and therefore require more oxygen. In a healthy heart this is not a problem, because the vessels dilate and the heart receives more oxygenated blood on call. However, when the heart is diseased, this dilation does not take place.

A common disease that causes this problem is **arteriosclerosis**, more commonly called hardening of the arteries, in which the artery walls become thickened and inelastic. **Atherosclerosis** is the form of arteriosclerosis that affects the coronary arteries and causes coronary artery disease. With this condition, the walls of the coronary arteries become thick and hard. The process is usually gradual and may take years to develop. The process begins with small deposits in the arteries that with time increase in size and cause a narrowing of the arteries. Calcification follows, and eventually the diameter of the artery becomes dangerously small.

The degree of this narrowing and the severity of the coronary artery disease determine the adverse effects the patient experiences. For example, with a narrowing of the arteries, the patient may experience angina pectoris. However, if the artery is extremely narrow or perhaps even occluded, myocardial infarction may occur.

This disease can also progress. The patient may have experienced angina for a period of time; then, as the disease increases in severity, the patient may experience a myocardial infarction.

ANGINA PECTORIS

Angina pectoris is a Latin phrase that means a "strangling of the chest."

Angina is characterized by episodes of pain when the heart experiences oxygen deficiency. This oxygen deficiency may be caused by conditions that result in decreased blood flow to the heart, decreased capacity of the blood to carry oxygen, or increased workload in the heart.

In addition, some cases of angina may be the first sign of atherosclerotic disease of the coronary arteries.

Signs and Symptoms

The most common symptom of angina is pain, usually in the substernal area of the chest, although it can be located anywhere in the chest from the **epigastrium** to the base of the neck. That the pain may spread to the jaw and teeth should be of some concern to the dental team. In these situations it is not unusual for even an edentulous patient to consult a dentist with continuous jaw pain. Some patients may describe the condition as a pressure or tightness in the chest rather than as actual pain.

The duration of the pain associated with angina is just as important as the location. An angina episode usually lasts three to five minutes if the precipitating factors are removed. If the factors are not removed, the episode may last up to forty minutes. If the episode continues much longer, the possibility of a myocardial infarction should be considered.

During an attack, the patient usually remains motionless in an attempt to alleviate the pain. In most cases the pain ceases within minutes, and the patient may continue activity. However, if the patient does not stop activity at least for a short period, the pain worsens until it becomes almost unbearable. On the other hand, in a few patients the pain may stop without cessation of the physical activity. This "second-wind syndrome" is possible because the collateral channels may start to function, which decreases myocardial hypoxia.

The physical signs in an angina attack are usually not very reliable. Appearance may remain relatively normal, or the patient may appear pale with cold and clammy skin. The pulse rate and blood pressure may increase slightly before or coincidentally with the onset of an angina attack. The patient may also experience a feeling of impending doom.

EMERGENCY BASICS

Signs and Symptoms of Angina

- Substernal chest pain
- Patient remains motionless
- Normal appearance or paleness
- Increase in pulse rate
- Increase in blood pressure
- Cold, clammy skin
- Feeling of impending doom

Classifications of Angina

Angina pectoris is most often classed as either stable or unstable. Pain from stable angina usually occurs as a result of physical exertion or emotional upset. Stable angina usually does not alter in frequency, duration, or intensity within a sixty-day period, whereas unstable angina changes. Unstable angina is unpredictable in regard to cause, with episodes occurring even at rest. Attacks often increase in frequency, severity, and duration. Attacks that were once controlled by **nitroglycerin** may require a higher dosage or become completely immune to its effects.

PRECIPITATING FACTORS OF ANGINA EPISODES

Classically, angina occurs following physical exertion or emotional stress. Eating or drinking something cold may also trigger an attack. Other activities that may bring on an attack are bathing, dressing, or sex. The amount of stress necessary to cause an attack can vary from time to time, and an angina episode may occur at any time of day or night. A person may experience an attack immediately after going to bed as a result of the effort used to undress or bathe or on waking in the morning after disturbing dreams.

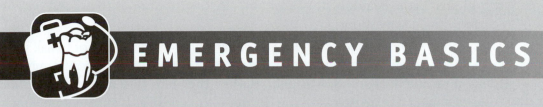

EMERGENCY BASICS

Comparison of Stable and Unstable Angina

Stable Angina
1. Pain result of physical or emotional stress
2. No alteration in duration, frequency, or intensity
3. Controlled with nitroglycerin

Unstable Angina
1. Pain may occur even at rest
2. Often increases in duration, frequency, or intensity
3. May require increase in dosage of nitroglycerin, or nitroglycerin may have no effect

Diagnosis

If the patient experiences chest pain while in the dental office, the dentist must attempt to determine the cause. The first course of action is to recheck the patient's medical history for any notations of angina or other cardiac

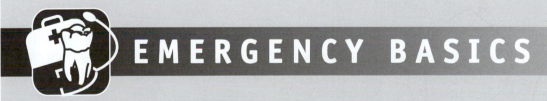

EMERGENCY BASICS

Precipitating Factors of Angina Episodes

1. Physical exertion
2. Emotional stress
3. Eating or drinking cold foods
4. Dressing
5. Bathing
6. Sexual activity
7. Disturbing dreams

problems. If the health history is of no help, one solution is to ask the patient certain crucial questions:

1. *What type of discomfort are you experiencing?* It is best not to ask what type of pain the patient is experiencing because some people may not describe the condition as pain. Rather, they may describe the condition as being like a vise clamping down on the chest or like someone standing on the chest. Others may describe the condition as a dull, burning sensation. If the patient describes a sharp or knifelike pain, the condition is probably not angina pectoris.

2. *Describe the location of your discomfort.* Angina pectoris pain is not usually well localized. If the patient can point to one small area where the pain is occurring, the problem is most likely not angina. Most often angina is felt in the substernal area in the middle of the chest. The pain may radiate down either or both arms and may cause a feeling of numbness. The pain may also radiate to the neck or jaw.

3. *How long did your discomfort last?* Angina pain is usually steady, with very little change in intensity, and may last from a minute to several hours. However, the longer the pain lasts, the greater the chances of the patient experiencing a myocardial infarction. Pain that fluctuates or lasts only a few seconds is usually not angina.

4. *What preceded the discomfort?* Angina pain is usually brought on by physical exertion or emotional stress. Exposure to cold weather or eating a large meal may also be a precipitating factor. It is beneficial for the dental team to be aware of the precipitating factors to prevent a recurrence of the attack.

5. *What provided relief from your discomfort?* If relief comes after resting for a few minutes, taking nitroglycerin, or both, the condition is most likely angina. Remember, however, that this is a very tricky situation, since some other serious heart conditions may mimic these symptoms.

Some of these questions may not be appropriate if the patient is experiencing an angina episode. Since the basic symptoms of most heart conditions are very similar, the emergency diagnosis may depend on the patient's response to certain treatment. For example, if the patient is treated with nitroglycerin and the pain is not relieved, the condition may be myocardial infarction rather than angina.

Treatment

Once the dentist has diagnosed the patient's condition as angina pectoris, the goal of treatment must be to reduce the demand of the heart muscle for oxygen. This is achieved by these steps:

1. Remain calm. It is vital that the patient have confidence in your ability to manage the situation. This is especially important if this is the first time the patient has experienced an angina attack. The dental team should alleviate as much anxiety as possible.
2. Stop all dental treatment. Be sure to remove all items from the patient's mouth. Also be sure to remove from the patient's sight all items that may have been causing concern or anxiety, such as syringes.
3. Position the patient. Place the patient in whatever position is most comfortable. Loosen all tight clothing such as neckties or belts.
4. Administer nitroglycerin. Ask patients who have reported a medical history of angina if they have their nitroglycerin with them. If they do, be sure and place the medication within easy reach. Most emergency kits contain nitroglycerin, but it is best that patients administer their own, since the dosage has been determined to meet their needs. The nitroglycerin should be placed sublingually and allowed to dissolve.
5. Administer oxygen. Since the patient is suffering from a lack of oxygenated blood reaching the heart, administering oxygen makes the patient more comfortable.

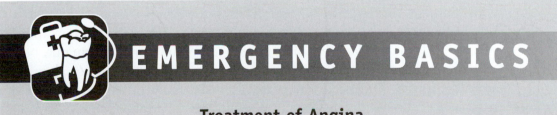

EMERGENCY BASICS

Treatment of Angina

1. Remain calm
2. Stop dental treatment
3. Position patient
4. Administer nitroglycerin
5. Administer oxygen
6. Administer second dose of nitroglycerin if needed, or amyl nitrite
7. Summon medical assistance if necessary

6. If the angina is not relived by the first dose of nitroglycerin, a second dose may be administered.

7. If nitroglycerin is not available, **amyl nitrite** may be administered. However, in some instances some unpleasant side effects are associated with this drug, so administer it only if nitroglycerin is not available.

8. If the treatment described is unsuccessful in relieving the patient's symptoms, the dental team should assume the patient is experiencing myocardial infarction rather than angina and treat accordingly.

Nitroglycerin

Nitroglycerin is a coronary vasodilator prescribed for the prevention or relief of angina. Its function is to help dilate the coronary arteries to allow more oxygenated blood to reach the heart. Sublingual nitroglycerin has become the accepted drug for the relief of angina episodes because of its rapid action. On the average, effects of nitroglycerin are noticeable within 90 seconds after sublingual administration of the correct dose. Nitroglycerin is administered sublingually because it can be rapidly absorbed through the buccal mucosa.

Other forms of nitroglycerin are more commonly used in the prophylactic treatment of angina. Some patients may use an ointment form of nitroglycerin, which they place on the chest before participating in a physical activity they feel may trigger an attack.

Individual sensitivity to nitroglycerin varies, so a physician will determine the correct dose for each individual. For this reason, it is important to allow patients to administer their own nitroglycerin if possible.

Nitroglycerin should improve the patient's condition within about a minute and a half. However, if it is not effective, the nitroglycerin may be old and therefore not longer effective (which is why nitroglycerin should be stored in its original bottle with the cap tightly sealed). Also, the atherosclerosis may be so severe that the drug is no longer effective and other medication may be needed.

Two common side effects are associated with the use of nitroglycerin. First, **orthostatic hypotension** can occur (it may be corrected with dose adjustments). Second, severe headaches may result when nitroglycerin administration is first started. Most clinicians have observed the disappearance of these initial headaches during the continued administration of the nitroglycerin.

Although nitroglycerin alone allows most angina sufferers to lead normal lives, in some cases multiple drugs such as beta blocks may also be required.

MYOCARDIAL INFARCTION

As mentioned earlier, atherosclerosis causes a narrowing of the coronary vessels. When this condition is not severe, angina usually occurs. However, when there is a significant narrowing or a blockage of the coronary arteries, a condition known as *myocardial infarction* may occur. Myocardial infarction is included in the section with angina because in some cases angina attacks may advance to myocardial infarction. On the other hand, myocardial infarction may occur in a patient who has never experienced an angina episode.

Myocardial infarction is a condition that occurs when a portion of the myocardium dies as a result of oxygen starvation caused by the narrowing or complete blockage of the artery that supplies that area with blood.

The condition may be created by any problem that causes an inadequate supply of oxygenated blood to reach the myocardium, a very common cause being atherosclerosis.

Signs and Symptoms

The pain associated with myocardial infarction most often occurs when the patient is at rest. Most victims, when questioned after the attack, report that they experienced angina-type pain hours to days prior to the myocardial infarction. The compressing, squeezing pain usually begins in the substernal area and then spreads to other areas. The pain associated with myocardial infarction may vary in degree from severe to almost nonexistent. It may last for 30 minutes or may even continue until analgesic medication is administered. This pain is not relieved by nitroglycerin.

Furthermore, the patient may have cold and clammy skin, vomiting, nausea, dizziness, or hypotension and may exhibit shortness of breath, sweating, weakness, extreme fatigue, anxiety, and a feeling of impending doom.

In the final stages the patient may pass through stupor, coma, and ultimately death.

Treatment

1. Remain calm. As with any emergency situation, it is important that the patient have confidence in your ability.

EMERGENCY BASICS

Signs and Symptoms of Myocardial Infarction

- Pain usually occurs at rest
- Compressing, squeezing pain beginning in substernal area and spreading
- Severity of pain varies
- Pain is not relieved by nitroglycerin
- Cold, clammy skin
- Vomiting
- Nausea
- Sweating
- Weakness or extreme fatigue
- Feeling of impending doom

2. Stop all dental treatment. Be sure to remove all materials and equipment from in and around the patient's mouth.

3. Administer nitroglycerin. Remember that several heart conditions present similar symptoms. This aids in diagnosis because nitroglycerin does not relieve the pain of myocardial infarction.

4. Summon medical assistance. A person experiencing a myocardial infarction requires hospital care.

5. Keep the patient as quiet and calm as possible. Some patients suffering myocardial infarction may move about in an effort to get comfortable. However, it is of utmost importance to try to keep the patient from placing any additional stress or strain on the heart.

6. Position the patient. Most myocardial infarction victims are most comfortable in a seated position.

7. Provide oxygen. This helps the patient rest more comfortably.

8. Assist patients in taking their medication if they are under a doctor's care.

9. Be prepared for any complication, including cardiac arrest.

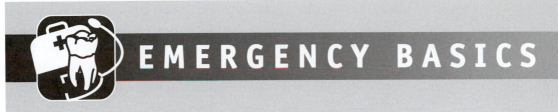

Treatment of Myocardial Infarction

1. Stop dental treatment
2. Administer nitroglycerin
3. Summon medical assistance if nitroglycerin does not relieve pain
4. Keep patient quiet and calm
5. Position patient
6. Provide oxygen
7. Be prepared to perform CPR

DIFFERENCES BETWEEN ANGINA AND MYOCARDIAL INFARCTION

1. The pain associated with myocardial infarction is usually greater in severity and duration than with angina.
2. Myocardial infarction pain occurs in the absence of physical exertion or emotional stress.
3. The myocardial infarction patient continues to move about trying to find a comfortable position, whereas the angina patient remains motionless.

Stress

Emotional tension plays a major role as a precipitating factor of angina. In addition, chest discomfort from a stressful situation tends to last longer than that caused by physical exertion because emotions are not as easy to control as physical activity.

Prevention

The patient experiencing angina, especially the first time, is very frightened and upset. Most associate the chest discomfort with impending death, primarily because most people know someone who has died from a heart problem. This concern and fear increases the need for oxygen going to the heart and therefore has a tendency to worsen the condition. The dental team must work to relieve this fear. This may be accomplished by prompt treatment to relieve the chest discomfort, maintaining control of the situation, and reassuring the patient.

It is always better to try to prevent an angina attack from occurring in the dental office than to have to treat an episode, because an angina attack can lead to myocardial infarction and even to death. Prevention is accomplished by being aware of the patient's medical history and taking steps to alleviate stress from the dental visit.

With all dental patients, it is important to try to make the visit pain-free, but this is especially important with the patient with a history of coronary problems. Pain tends to cause stress, which will aggravate a heart condition and possibly trigger an attack.

It may also be necessary to limit the length of the dental appointment for heart patients, since the stress placed on such patients by a long appointment may also trigger an attack.

SUMMARY

Heart disease is the leading cause of death in the United States today and is therefore a possible emergency the dental team may have to deal with. Angina is a condition most patients are aware that they have and will note on the health history. In these situations, the dental team should do everything possible to alleviate undue stress, which may trigger an angina episode. It is certainly more beneficial to prevent an angina attack from occurring than to treat it once it happens. Angina, allowed to progress without proper treatment, may escalate to myocardial infarction. At the same time, myocardial infarction can occur without the patient having a history of angina. The dental team should try to prevent as much stress as possible and then be aware of the signs, symptoms, and treatment for a cardiac emergency in case it occurs while the patient is in the dental office.

REFERENCES

Altschule, Mark D. "The Etiology of Atherosclerosis." *Medical Clinics of North America* 58 (March 1974).

Altschule, Mark D. "Physiology in Acute Myocardial Infarction." *Medical Clinics of North America* 58 (March 1974).

Andreoli, Kathleen Gaynor. *Comprehensive Cardiac Care*. 5th ed. St. Louis: Mosby, 1983.

Chiamvimonat, V., and Sternberg, L., "Coronary artery disease in women." *Canadian Family Physician*, December 1998.

Cohn, Peter F., and Richard Gorlin. "Physiologic and Clinical Actions of Nitroglycerin." *Medical Clinics of North American 58* (March 1974).

Cosby, Richard S. "Late Complications of Myocardial Infarction." *Journal of the American Medical Association* (October 11, 1976).

Dalager-Pedersen S., Ravn, H. B., & Falk, E. "Atherosclerosis and acute coronary events." *American Journal of Cardiology*, November 26, 1998.

Eliot, Robert S., and Alan D. Forker. "Emotional Stress and Cardiac Disease." *Journal of the American Medical Association* (November 15, 1976).

Farkouh, M.E., et al. "A clinical trial of a chest-pain observation unit for patients with unstable angina." *The New England Journal of Medicine*. December 24, 1998.

Frank, Martin J. "What to Do for the Patient with Unstable Angina." *Consultant* (January 1979).

Jacob, Stanley W. *Structure and Function in Man*. 2nd ed. Philadelphia: Saunders, 1970.

McGregor, Maurice. "Pathogenesis of Angina Pectoris and Role of Nitrates in Relief of Myocardial Ischemia." *The American Journal of Medicine* (June 27, 1983).

McSweeney, J.C. "Women's narratives: Evolving symptoms of myocardial infarction." *Journal of Women and Aging, 10* (2), 1998.

Reichek, Nathaniel. "Role of Nitroglycerin in Effort Angina." *The American Journal of Medicine* (June 27, 1983).

Riseman, Joseph E. F. "Diagnosis of Angina Pectoris at the Present Time." *Medical Clinics of North America 58* (March 1974).

Segal, Bernard L. "Clinical Recognition of Angina Pectoris." *Geriatrics* (November 1979).

Segal, Bernard L. "Unstable Angina Pectoris: Therapeutic Choices." *Hospital Practice* (July 1980).

Tannenbaum, Renee P. "Angina Pectoris: How to Recognize It, How to Manage It." *Nursing 81* (September 1981).

REVIEW QUESTIONS

MULTIPLE CHOICE

1. The layer of the wall of the heart that gives the heart the ability to contract is the:
   a. epicardium
   b. myocardium
   c. endocardium
   d. pericardium

2. Which of the following is not a characteristic of unstable angina?
   a. episodes may occur at rest
   b. no alteration in frequency
   c. may require higher dose of nitroglycerin
   d. episodes often increase in intensity and duration

3. Which of the following is a precipitating factor of angina?
   a. drinking a cold drink
   b. sexual activity
   c. walking
   d. all the above

4. When treating a patient experiencing an angina attack, it is best to give the patient her own nitroglycerin because:
   a. the office supply of nitroglycerin should be saved for patients who are not taking nitroglycerin.
   b. you will be assured that the nitroglycerin is not expired
   c. the doses will be adjusted for that particular event
   d. none of the above

5. If all the normal treatment for angina does not relieve the pain, the dental team should assume that the patient is suffering from:
   a. cerebrovascular accident
   b. cardiac arrest
   c. respiratory distress
   d. myocardial infarction

6. The coronary vasodilator most commonly used to treat angina is:
   a. insulin
   b. nitroglycerin
   c. bronchodilator
   d. epinephrine

7. Which of the following is not a sign or symptom of myocardial infarction?
   a. most often occurs following physical exertion or emotional stress
   b. compressing, squeezing pain in the substernal area
   c. may last in duration for 30 minutes or more
   d. feeling of impending doom

8. When positioning the myocardial infarction patient, it is best to place the patient in a _____ position.
   a. supine
   b. seated
   c. standing
   d. none of the above

9. The syndrome characterized by episodes of pain when the heart experiences oxygen deficiency is:
   a. cardiac arrest
   b. myocardial infarction
   c. pulmonary edema
   d. none of the above

10. Which of the following is a sign or symptom of angina?
    a. substernal chest pain
    b. patient remains motionless
    c. increase in blood pressure
    d. all the above

TRUE OR FALSE

T 1. Atherosclerosis is the form of arteriosclerosis that affects the coronary arteries and causes coronary artery disease.

T 2. The amount of stress necessary to cause an angina attack can vary from time to time.

T 3. The most common symptom of angina is pain.

F 4. During an angina attack, the patient moves about a great deal in an effort to get comfortable.

T 5. Nitroglycerin should be stored in its original bottle with the cap tightly sealed.

F 6. Myocardial infarction pain does not occur in the absence of physical exertion or emotional stress.

T 7. Nitroglycerin should be placed sublingually and allowed to dissolve.

T 8. Orthostatic hypotension and headache are common side effects of nitroglycerin.

F 9. Angina pectoris never advances to myocardial infarction.

F 10. Pain associated with myocardial infarction is usually relieved by nitroglycerin.

■ CASE STUDY

Bob Tatum, 44 years old, reported on the health history that he has been experiencing angina attacks for two years. He has his nitroglycerin with him. Tatum is in the office to have an amalgam placed in number 12. The dentist administers anesthesia and begins treatment. The patient becomes pale and starts to clutch at his chest. The dentist stops treatment and allows the patient to administer his own nitroglycerin. Tatum says his chest pain is usually not so severe. He tries to get up and move around in an effort to relieve the pain. After several minutes, the patient's pain still has not been relieved. The patient takes another dose of nitroglycerin, but the pain still does not stop.

QUESTIONS

1. Is the patient most likely suffering from angina or myocardial infarction?
2. What treatment should be followed after administering the second dose of nitroglycerin?
3. Should oxygen be administered to this patient? Why or why not?
4. What should the dental assistant be doing during this treatment?

11

Cardiopulmonary Resuscitation

KEY TERMS

Artificial respiration
Brachial artery
Cardiac arrest
Carotid artery
External compression
Gastric distention

Laryngectomy
Mandible
Pulse
Sternum
Stoma
Xiphoid process

OBJECTIVES

Upon completion of this chapter the student will be able to:

- Explain the ABCs of CPR
- Demonstrate how to determine consciousness
- Describe the technique for administering artificial respiration
- Demonstrate how to check the carotid pulse
- Explain the technique for administering external compressions

- Explain when CPR should be started and stopped
- Explain the technique of two-person CPR
- Explain how to open the airway in a child or infant
- Explain how to provide artificial respiration for infants and children
- Explain how to check an infant's pulse at the brachial artery
- Explain how to administer external compressions for infants and children
- Describe two of the dangers associated with administering CPR

The content of this chapter is intended as an overview of the CPR technique. All dental personnel should take a CPR course offered by the American Heart Association or the American Red Cross and become certified in the technique. This certification should then be renewed on a regular basis.

Also keep in mind that advances and modifications in techniques are constantly occurring. Dental auxiliaries should maintain current certification to ensure they are using the most up-to-date CPR techniques.

CARDIAC ARREST

Cardiac arrest exists when the circulation of blood either is absent or is inadequate to maintain life. Although cardiac arrest may be the end result of conditions such as angina or myocardial infarction, it may also occur by itself with no previous signs or coronary disease.

Cardiac arrest may present itself as one of these three conditions:

1. *Cardiovascular collapse.* The heart is still beating but is so weak that it cannot circulate the blood.
2. *Ventricular fibrillation.* Individual muscles beat independently rather than as a unit, which results in no blood being circulated.
3. *Cardiac standstill.* The heart has stopped beating.

In past decades, if a person experienced some form of cardiac arrest, the chances of survival prior to admittance to a hospital were remote. The technique of cardiopulmonary resuscitation was then devised, and these odds were improved. Cardiopulmonary resuscitation, more commonly known as CPR, consists of combining artificial respiration with external cardiac compressions in an attempt to force oxygenated blood throughout the body.

CPR is able to achieve its effects primarily because of the location of the heart. The heart is located between the **sternum** and thoracic spine and is surrounded on either side by the lungs and pericardium. As a result of this location, force applied to the lower sternum creates a pressure that drives the blood through the aorta and pulmonary artery. This blood is then oxygenated by combining artificial respiration with the compressions.

The greatest risk of death from heart attack occurs in the first two hours after the onset of symptoms. If the public is trained in CPR, heart attack victims can receive treatment immediately, which increases the chances of survival.

Since the inception of CPR, people within the medical community have argued about its benefits as well as its hazards. No matter what the arguments include, it has been proved that CPR can save lives. As a result of the number of people trained in CPR, between 100,000 and 200,000 American lives have been saved each year.

The biggest advantage of CPR is that it can provide immediate treatment for respiratory arrest or cardiac arrest without the need for any adjunct equipment or personnel.

TECHNIQUE

The technique of CPR is broken down into steps known as the ABCs of CPR. The A stands for AIRWAY opened, B for BREATHING restored, and C for CIRCULATION restored. These ABCs designate the order in which CPR must be performed.

When an unconscious patient is discovered—or if the dental patient loses consciousness—the presence or absence of breathing and circulation must be determined immediately. If breathing is absent, opening the airway and providing artificial respiration may be all that is needed. If circulation is also absent, external compression must be combined with artificial respiration, thus administering full CPR.

Determining Consciousness

When the endangered victim is discovered, the first step of treatment is to determine consciousness. (In most dental settings, this is not as difficult as in the unknown victim, because the dental patient is usually being observed when unconsciousness occurs.) This technique is performed by the rescuer tapping the patient firmly on the shoulder and shouting in the patient's ear, "Are you all right? Are you all right?" The rescuer must make sure the victim is unconscious and not asleep or in a drug-induced stupor.

Opening the Airway

Once the rescuer has determined that the victim is unconscious, it is necessary to open the airway. After opening the airway, if the patient is not breathing independently, the rescuer needs to breathe for the victim. These two steps combined constitute **artificial respiration**. These steps can and should be performed immediately.

When opening the airway, the rescuer should keep in mind that the tongue is the most common cause of airway obstruction in an unconscious victim. The victim who loses consciousness may also lose muscle tone, which may cause the tongue to drop to the back of the throat, blocking the airway. Consequently, to open the airway, a method that pulls the tongue away from the back of the throat must be used. This is best achieved by implementing a technique known as the head tilt/chin lift. To accomplish this, the rescuer places the hand closest to the patient's head on the forehead and gently tilts the head back. At the same time, the rescuer uses the hand closest to the patient's feet to lift the patient's chin by placing the fingers—not the thumb—under the bony part of the **mandible** at the chin and lifting the chin upward. This technique lifts the tongue away from the airway. Care must be taken not to close the patient's mouth completely or to put pressure on the soft tissues located under the chin.

Artificial Respiration

The rescuer should open the airway and then check to determine if spontaneous breathing is occurring. Once the airway is opened, the rescuer places an ear close to the victim's mouth. In this position the rescuer is able to look for the rise and fall of the chest, listen for air during exhalation, and feel for air against the cheek (Figure 11-1). Once the airway has been opened, the patient may begin to breathe spontaneously. If the victim is not breathing, the rescuer should administer artificial respiration.

To administer artificial respiration, the rescuer first seals the nose by pinching the victim's nostrils between the thumb and forefinger of the hand that was on the victim's forehead. Next, the rescuer takes a deep breath, opens her mouth very wide, and places it around the outside of the victim's mouth. If the rescuer's lips are placed on the inside of the victim's mouth, a good seal will not form and air will leak around the edges, preventing sufficient air from entering the victim's lungs. Once a good seal has formed, the rescuer blows air into the victim's mouth. During the ventilations, the rescuer should observe the victim to make sure sufficient oxygen is reaching the victim's lungs. This may be achieved by watching the rise and fall of the

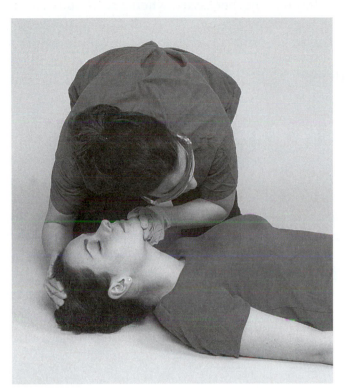

Figure 11-1 Checking for spontaneous breathing

chest, feeling slight resistance as the air enters the victim's lungs, and feeling the air escape during exhalation. (See Figure 11-1.)

If the rescuer is able to get air into the victim's lungs, the first breathing sequence should consist of two breaths with 1-1.5 seconds allowed for each breath. Each breath should be separate, allowing the lungs to deflate between each breath.

A rescuer unable to get air into the victim's lungs should reposition the airway and attempt to ventilate again. If it is still impossible to get air into the lungs, the rescuer must assume there is an airway obstruction and should follow the procedures covered in chapter 4.

Mouth-to-Nose Respiration

Some conditions may require that respiration be administered using a mouth-to-nose technique rather than a mouth-to-mouth technique. For example, this may be necessary when the mouth is damaged to such an extent that a good seal cannot be formed. If this technique is required, the rescuer should keep the head tilted back with the hand on the forehead and use the other hand to close the victim's mouth. The rescuer then makes a seal with the mouth around the victim's nose and administers the two slow breaths.

Mouth-to-Stoma Respiration

As treatment for certain conditions, some victims may have had a **laryngectomy**. This results in a **stoma**, or opening, that connects the trachea directly to an opening in the skin. In these situations it is necessary for the rescuer to administer ventilations directly to the victim's stoma. It is not necessary to open the airway because the stoma is at the bottom of the airway.

Gastric Distention

When the rescuer is administering artificial respiration, a condition known as **gastric distention** can occur. This condition is seen most frequently in children, although it can also occur in adults. Gastric distention usually occurs when the rescuer uses too much air to ventilate the victim or when the airway is partially or completely blocked, which forces air into the stomach rather than the lungs.

Severe gastric distention can be dangerous because it may cause regurgitation with the vomitus aspirated into the lungs, causing an obstruction. Furthermore, it can reduce the lung capacity if the distended stomach causes the diaphragm to be elevated.

Checking the Pulse

Cardiac arrest is recognized by the absence of a **pulse** in the large arteries. Once the rescuer has administered the two breaths, the next step is to determine if the victim has a pulse.

To achieve this, the rescuer maintains the open airway with the hand on the victim's forehead and uses the first two fingers of the other hand to check the victim's carotid pulse. The **carotid artery** is used to determine the presence of a pulse because it is accessible without removing any clothes, the rescuer is already positioned close to this area, and—most important—there may be a pulse in this artery even when the pulse in the periphery is absent. This artery is located by placing fingers on the victim's larynx and sliding them into the groove between the trachea and the muscles on the side of the neck. There is a carotid artery on either side of the neck; either may be used to check the pulse (Figure 11-2). When checking the pulse, the rescuer should never compress too hard, because the artery could be occluded.

The pulse should always be checked for at least five seconds but not more than ten seconds. It is important to wait at least five seconds because in some emergency situations the pulse may have slowed to such a point that it would not be palpable for at least five seconds. If a pulse is present, the rescuer continues to administer artificial respiration. If a pulse is not present, the rescuer activates the EMS system. This consists of instructing another member of the dental team or a bystander, depending on the circumstances, to call 911 or 0 for medical help. It is important to give exact directions to the location so that the emergency team can get to the patient quickly.

EXTERNAL COMPRESSION

Absence of pulse indicates that the heart is no longer supplying blood and must be replaced by external compression.

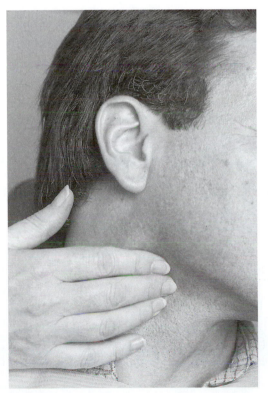

Figure 11-2 Location of carotid pulse

External compression consists of applying rhythmic pressure over the lower sternum, which raises the thoracic pressure and forces the blood out of the heart.

Chest compression must always be accompanied by artificial respiration because there must be some means of oxygenating the blood.

Before administering compression, the positioning of the patient is extremely important. The cardiac arrest victim must always be in the horizontal position. The external compressions are able to force blood throughout the body, but they are not powerful enough to overcome the forces of gravity in a person in any position other than horizontal.

In addition, the patient must be on a firm surface. Since the whole purpose of external compression is to squeeze the heart between the sternum and spine, if the patient is on a soft surface the force of the compression is absorbed. Contoured dental chairs are not recommended for performing compression. A dental patient who requires compression should be placed either on the floor or on a board placed between the patient and the chair.

Technique

Once the patient is properly positioned, external compression is administered following these steps:

1. The rescuer is positioned close to the patient's chest.
2. The rescuer must locate the proper hand position for administering the compressions by placing the index and middle finger of the hand closest to the victim's feet at the base of the victim's rib on the side closest to the rescuer.
3. The rescuer then slides the fingers up the rib cage to the area where the ribs meet the sternum.
4. The middle finger rests at this area with the index finger placed beside it. This technique is used to locate the lower portion of the sternum. The location is extremely important because if the hand position is too low, compression takes place over the **xiphoid process** rather than the lower sternum. If compressions are performed over the xiphoid process, it could be broken and the liver lacerated, and if compressions are too high they will be ineffective.
5. Once the lower part of the sternum is located, the heel of the hand closest to the patient's head is placed directly beside the index finger.
6. The first hand is then removed and placed on top of the hand resting on the sternum.

7. The fingers are interlocked, which helps keep the fingers off the chest during compression. Fingers pressing on the chest during compression can damage the ribs.

8. The rescuer's elbows are locked and the shoulders positioned over the hands. This way the compressions are performed by utilizing the rescuer's body weight rather than utilizing only the arm muscles. (See Figure 11-3.)

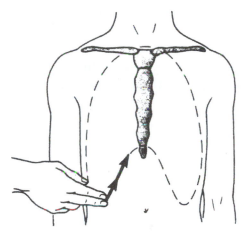

A. Trace along rib cage to notch

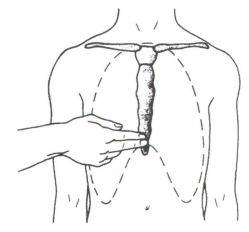

B. Place middle finger on notch with index finger beside it.

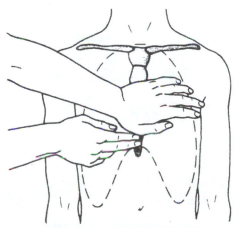

C. Measure by placing one hand beside the index finger of the other hand.

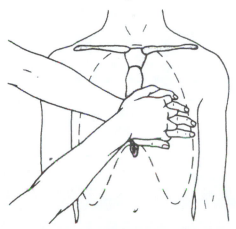

D. Lace fingers and keep them off the chest.

Figure 11-3 Hand positioning for external compressions

9. The size of the patient determines the depth the chest must be compressed to achieve effective compression. For an adult, the sternum is compressed approximately 1.5 to 2.0 inches. This depth is required to adequately force the blood out of the heart.

10. Immediately following the compression, the rescuer releases the sternum to allow the heart to refill. During this release, the hands are not removed from the chest, since correct hand position must not be lost.

11. Compressions should be smooth and rhythmic, with equal time spent on compression and release.

12. In one-person CPR, the rescuer gives 15 compressions in 9-11 seconds. The rescuer should administer these compressions by counting aloud: "1 and 2 and 3 ... and 14 and 15." The compression is made when the rescuer says the number, and the release is made when the rescuer says *and*.

13. After the 15th compression, the rescuer administers two full slow breaths and then returns to the chest, locates the correct hand position, and gives 15 more compressions.

14. After three or four sequences of 15 compressions and two breaths, the rescuer checks the carotid pulse. If there is a pulse and breathing the rescuer monitors the patient. If there is no pulse, the rescuer continues CPR.

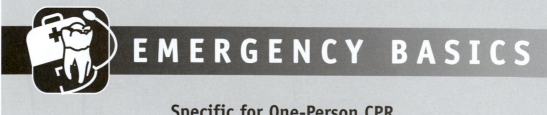

EMERGENCY BASICS

Specific for One-Person CPR

Hand position: 2 hands
Rates: 15 compressions, 2 breaths
Depth: 1.5"-2.0"

Starting and Stopping CPR

To achieve the greatest benefits, CPR should be started immediately upon recognition of cardiac arrest. Some degree of brain damage may occur if the

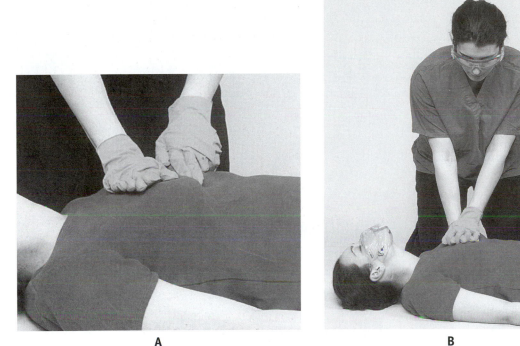

A   B

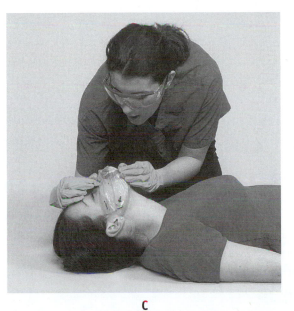

C

Figure 11-4 (A) Tilt back head and lift chin. Locate hand on the breastbone two inches above xiphoid process. (B) Position your shoulders over your hands and compress the chest fifteen times. (C) Give two slow breaths, holding nose.

brain is deprived of oxygen for more than six minutes; if CPR is not started within this time, it is unlikely that the patient will be restored to previous CNS levels. However, the victim should receive the benefit of the doubt and the rescuer should attempt CPR.

Once CPR has been started in the absence of a physician, it should be continued until one of the following conditions is met:

1. The victim recovers.
2. CPR efforts are transferred to another qualified person trained in CPR.
3. A physician assume responsibility for the victim.
4. EMS personnel (EMTs or paramedics) assume responsibility for the victim.
5. The rescuer is exhausted and physically unable to continue CPR.

Two-Person CPR

The rates and rhythms previously covered apply to one-person CPR for adults. Although CPR can successfully be performed by one rescuer, it quickly becomes physically exhausting when a single person must carry out compressions and respirations. It is much more beneficial if two people can work together to perform CPR. Two-person CPR consists of one person administering compression while the second person administers respiration.

If two rescuers begin CPR together, one person is positioned at the victim's chest and is responsible for administering compression while the second person is positioned at the head and is responsible for maintaining an open airway and providing respiration.

There may be situations when one person is alone and must begin CPR. A second person can join the first rescuer on arrival.

CPR FOR INFANTS AND CHILDREN

Cardiac arrest does not occur very often in infants or children. Nevertheless, there may be some emergency situations when cardiac arrest occurs and CPR is required. The basic principles of CPR are the same for adults, infants, and children. However, the anatomical differences in size require a few adjustments in techniques.

Categorizing Infants and Children

For purposes of CPR, an infant is considered anyone under one year of age. A child is anyone between one and eight years of age. Anyone over eight is treated as an adult. In some individuals where actual age is unknown, size may make it difficult to determine whether the individual should be treated as a child or an infant. CPR should not be delayed in an effort to determine if the victim is a child or an infant. A slight error one way or the other will not cause a major problem.

Determining Consciousness in the Infant or Child

When the child or infant victim is discovered, it is necessary to first determine consciousness. The tap-and-shout method discussed for adults is appropriate for the child. A slightly different technique may be more beneficial with the infant. It is sometimes difficult to tap the infant victim with enough force to assume unconsciousness while still being gentle enough to prevent injury. Therefore, to determine consciousness in the infant, the rescuer should thump the bottom of the infant's foot while shouting the baby's name, if it is known. If there is no response to these stimuli, the rescuer should assume the infant is unconscious.

Positioning the Victim

Once the rescuer determines that the victim is unconscious, the next step is to position the victim. Whether a child or an infant, the victim should be placed supine on a hard flat surface. When dealing with an infant, better access may be provided by placing the infant on a table or countertop rather than on the floor.

Opening the Airway

After the victim is properly positioned, the rescuer opens the airway. For the infant or child, the head tilt/chin lift technique may be used. The technique should be performed as for adults. The only change is that it is extremely important not to overextend the child's or infant's neck when tilting the head. This could possibly damage the neck as well as close the airway instead of opening it.

Checking for Air Exchange

The rescuer must then check to see if the infant or child or breathing. This can be done by placing an ear close to the victim's mouth, looking for the rise and fall of the chest, listening for air exchange, and feeling for air against the cheek.

Breathing

If the victim is not breathing, the rescuer must provide artificial respiration, a technique that varies for infants and for children.

Child

If the child is large enough for the rescuer to form a good seal around the mouth, the air may be provided using the same techniques as with the adult.

Infant

In the case of an infant or very small child, the rescuer needs to form a seal by placing the mouth over the infant's mouth and nose (Figure 11-6).

Once a sufficient seal is achieved by covering the victim's mouth or mouth and nose, the rescuer should administer two full slow breaths. Remember that the lungs of an infant or child are smaller than an adult's, and the amount of air administered must be adjusted according to the size of the child. However, the air passages of the infant and child are also small-

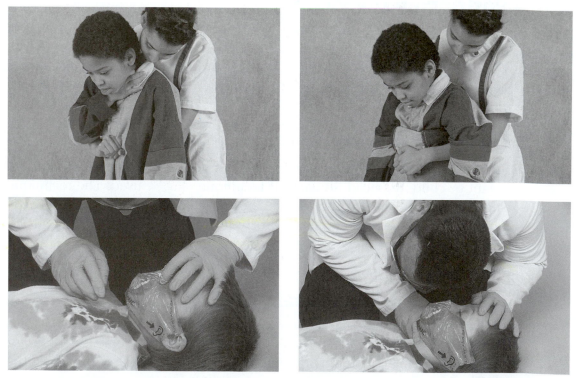

Figure 11-5 Artificial respiration for a child

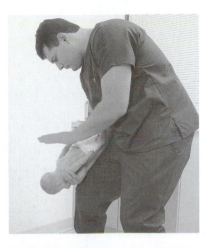
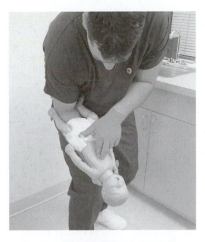
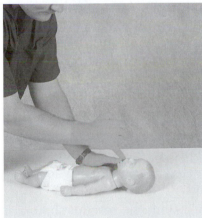
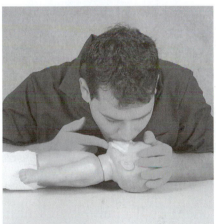
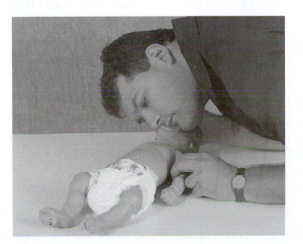

Figure 11-6 Artificial respiration for an infant

er and as a result provide more resistance when the rescuer attempts to blow air into the victim's lungs. The rescuer should not be afraid to use some force to get air into the lungs.

If the rescuer is unable to get air into the victim's lungs, the airway should be reopened and an attempt made to ventilate again. If it is still impossible to get air into the victim's lungs, the rescuer should assume there is an airway obstruction and proceed as described in chapter 4.

On the other hand, if air flows easily into the victim's lungs, the rescuer should provide the two full slow breaths and proceed to the next step.

Checking the Pulse

The next step in the CPR sequence is to check the infant or child's pulse. In a child, the presence of a pulse can be determined by palpating the carotid artery. In an infant, however, it is sometimes difficult or even impossible to palpate the carotid artery. This is difficult because an infant usually has a very short, fat neck that prevents access to the carotid artery.

It is best to check the infant's pulse by palpating the **brachial artery**. The brachial artery is located on the inside of the arm midway between the elbow and the shoulder. To palpate this pulse, the rescuer places the thumb on the outside of the victim's arm and the index and middle finger over the brachial artery and presses, lightly. Some people have difficulty locating this pulse, and extra practice should be directed to this area when mastering CPR skills.

If a pulse is present but breathing is absent, the rescuer should provide artificial respirations only, utilizing the following rates:

Infant: one puff every three seconds

Child: one breath every four seconds

If the brachial or carotid artery is palpated and there is no pulse the rescuer must provide external compressions.

The techniques for administering external compressions are different for infants and children. Each will be covered separately.

External Compressions

Child

When administering compressions for a child, the first step is to locate the correct hand position, achieved the same way as for adults.

The bone structure of a child is more fragile than that of an adult, so the same amount of force is not needed to compress the sternum. Only the heel of one hand is used to compress the sternum 1.0 to 1.5 inches.

Since a child's heart rate is faster than that of an adult, a compression rate of 80-100 per minute or 5 compressions every 3-4 seconds should be implemented. This is counted as "1 and 2 and 3 and 4 and 5 and...." Then the rescuer administers one breath. After three or four cycles, the pulse should be checked.

Infant

An infant's heart is located considerably higher in the chest than an adult's; the hand position for an infant is located at the midsternum right between the two nipples.

The bone structure of an infant is even more delicate than a child's. Therefore only the index and middle fingers of one hand are used to compress the midsternum 0.5-1 inch.

The heart rate of an infant is very fast, so the compressions must be much faster, at a rate of 100 compressions per minute, or 5 compressions in 3 seconds or less. This should be counted by the rescuer as "1, 2, 3, 4, 5...." After the fifth count, the rescuer administers one puff.

Unlike CPR for an adult, the rates remain the same for two-person CPR in infants and children. Furthermore, there is no set pattern for switching positions because the exertion required in two-person CPR is minimal.

DANGERS OF CPR

Because of the location of the ribs, sternum, and other organs, as well as the force required to perform CPR, injuries to the patient may occur. Incorrect hand position or excessive force can result in broken ribs. Placing the hands too low on the sternum and compressing the xiphoid process can lacerate the liver. Any of these factors can cause major problems to the victim, but should never cause the rescuer to hesitate beginning CPR.

SUMMARY

Thousands of Americans die from cardiac arrest each year. Some of these deaths occur in the dental office. By mastering the skills of CPR, the auxiliary puts forth a concerted effort to save lives both in the dental setting an in everyday life.

REFERENCES

Falk, Jay L., Eric Rackow, Brian Kaufman, and Max Harry Weil. "Cardiopulmonary Resuscitation: An Update." *Hospital Medicine* (January 1984).

Lonergan, James H. Joan Z. Youngberg, and Joel A. Kaplan. "Cardiopulmonary Resuscitation: Physical Stress on the Rescuer." *Critical Care Medicine 9* (November 1981).

Luce, John M., Jeffrey M. Cary, Brian K. Ross, Bruce H. Culver, and John Butler. "New Developments in Cardiopulmonary Resuscitation." *Journal of the American Medical Association, 244* (September 19, 1980).

Ludwig, Stephen, Robert G. Kettrick, and Margot Parker. "Pediatric Cardiopulmonary Resuscitation." *Clinical Pediatrics, 23* (February 1984).

"Standards and Guidelines for Cardiopulmonary Resuscitation and Emergency Cardiac Care." *Journal of the American Medical Association 244* (August 1, 1980).

"When Push Comes to Harm in CPR." *Emergency Medicine* (August 15, 1984).

REVIEW QUESTIONS

MULTIPLE CHOICE

1. Which of the following components comprise CPR?
   1. artificial respiration
   2. external compression
   3. checking blood pressure
   4. administering nitroglycerin
      a. 1, 2, 3
      b. 2, 3
      c. 1, 2
      d. 3, 4

2. Put the following steps of CPR in the correct order:
   1. administer two quick breaths
   2. administer external compressions
   3. open airway
   4. check pulse
      a. 1, 2, 3, 4
      b. 3, 1, 4, 2
      c. 4, 2, 3, 1
      d. 2, 1, 3, 4

3. Which of the following techniques should be used to administer ventilations to the laryngectomy victim?
   a. mouth-to-stoma
   b. mouth-to-mouth
   c. mouth-to-nose
   d. none of the above

4. When performing CPR on an adult, the _____ artery should be checked to determine the presence of a pulse.
   a. brachial
   b. radial
   c. femoral
   d. carotid

5. For an adult, external compressions should be administered:
   a. at midsternum
   b. over the xiphoid process
   c. over the lower half of the sternum
   d. none of the above

6. On an adult the sternum should be compressed:
   a. 0.5"-1.0"
   b. 2.0"-2.5"
   c. 1.0"-1.5"
   d. 1.5"-2.0"

7. On an adult the ratio of compressions to breaths is:
    a. 15 compressions: 2 breaths
    b. 5 compressions: 2 breaths
    c. 15 compressions: 1 breath
    d. none of the above

8. When checking the pulse on an infant, the _____ artery should be used.
    a. brachial
    b. femoral
    c. carotid
    d. radial

9. On a child the sternum should be compressed:
    a. 1.5"-2.0"
    b. 0.5"-1.0"
    c. 1.0"-1.5"
    d. 2.0"-2.5"

10. When administering compressions for an infant the rescuer should use:
    a. both hands interlocked
    b. the index and middle fingers of one hand
    c. the heel of one hand
    d. none of the above

TRUE OR FALSE

1. The biggest advantage of CPR is that is can be started immediately without any additional equipment or personnel.
2. The jaw-thrust technique should be used to open the airway if it is suspected that the victim may have a neck injury.
3. Gastric distention will never cause any problems for the victim.
4. For an infant the correct hand position is determined by following the ribs up to the lower part of the sternum.
5. When administering artificial respiration for a laryngectomy victim, the rescuer will administer respirations over the victim's mouth and nose.
6. For an adult, compressions and respirations are administered at a rate of 15:2.

7. Once CPR has been started, the rescuer may stop if he or she feels that the victim is not responding.
8. During two-person CPR, one rescuer provides artificial respirations while the other rescuer provides compressions.
9. The tap-and-shout method may be used on a child to determine consciousness.
10. There are no dangers to the victim from CPR.

■ CASE STUDY

Bill Watts, 40 and in good general health, has come to the dental office for his regular six-month checkup. While the appointment is in progress, Bill begins to complain of a tightness in his chest. He clutches his chest and then loses consciousness. The rescuer utilizes the head tilt/chin left technique to open the airway. The rescuer then checks for breathing and determines that Bill is not breathing. The rescuer gives one breath and then locates the brachial artery to determine if the victim has a pulse. No pulse is found, so the rescuer telephones the rescue squad for help. Next, the rescuer locates the lower half of the sternum and uses the heel of one hand to compress the sternum 1.5 to 2.0 inches. The rescuer administers 15 compressions, then returns to the victim's head and administers two breaths. After six to eight cycles, the rescuer checks the pulse. After 10 or 12 cycles the rescuer decides the patient is not responding and stops CPR.

QUESTIONS

1. List all the errors in this procedure.
2. For each error listed, explain what technique should have been performed.

12

Cerebrovascular Accident

KEY TERMS

Aneurysm
Cranium
Edema
Embolism
Hemiplegia

Hemorrhage
Hypertension
Ischemia
Thrombosis

OBJECTIVES

Upon completion of this chapter the student will be able to:

- Define cerebrovascular accident
- List the predisposing factors of a CVA
- Define the different classifications of a CVA
- List the signs and symptoms of a CVA
- Describe the treatment of a CVA

A cerebrovascular accident, also known as a CVA or stroke, is defined as a specific neurologic deficit that occurs suddenly as a result of vascular disease of a hemorrhagic or ischemic nature. The extent of the deficit depends on both the area of the brain involved and the cause of the deficit.

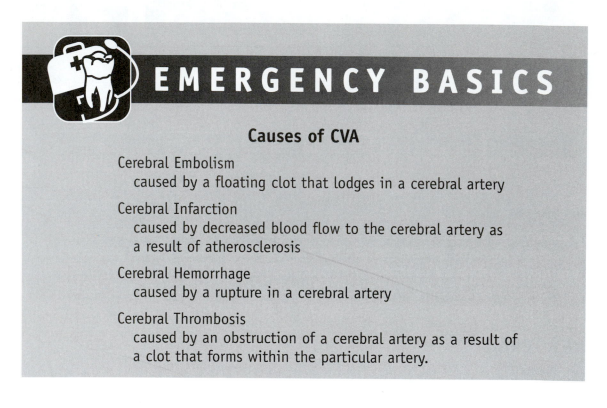

EMERGENCY BASICS

Causes of CVA

Cerebral Embolism
   caused by a floating clot that lodges in a cerebral artery

Cerebral Infarction
   caused by decreased blood flow to the cerebral artery as a result of atherosclerosis

Cerebral Hemorrhage
   caused by a rupture in a cerebral artery

Cerebral Thrombosis
   caused by an obstruction of a cerebral artery as a result of a clot that forms within the particular artery.

CLASSIFICATIONS

CVAs are classified according to cause. The causes of CVAs can be divided into the following categories: cerebral **embolism**, cerebral infarction, cerebral **hemorrhage**, and cerebral **thrombosis**. The signs and symptoms associated with each cause are similar, as is the treatment. Each type is discussed separately.

TRANSIENT ISCHEMIC ATTACK

A transient ischemic attack (TIA) is a neurologic deficit that lasts for a short period of time. Although a TIA is not an actual stroke, it is included in the classification of a CVA because it is so similar. The relationship between a TIA and a CVA is very similar to that of angina and myocardial infarction.

Sometimes it is difficult to determine whether the patient is suffering from a CVA or from a TIA. The best way to make a determination is by the duration of the episode. The TIA lasts only a few minutes and then the signs and symptoms cease, whereas the signs and symptoms of a true CVA do not regress.

Always remember too that a TIA has the potential to advance to a severe CVA. Whether a TIA advances to a complete stroke usually depends on the underlying cause of the TIA. If this cause is resolved, a complete stroke will not occur.

The clinical manifestations of a TIA vary according to the area of the brain affected. However, most people suffering from a TIA experience some numbness or weakness in the extremities. This numbness is sometimes described by the patient as a "pins-and-needles" feeling. Consciousness is usually not impaired, but the patient may appear somewhat confused during the episode.

TIAs also play another important role in their relationship to a complete CVA. It has been found through very careful questioning of stroke victims that they usually experienced some episodes of TIA before they experienced the complete stroke.

The TIA does not usually present an emergency situation in the dental office. However, if the patient has a history of repeated TIAs, the dental team should realize that this patient has increased chances for experiencing a severe CVA.

CEREBRAL EMBOLISM

A cerebral *embolism* is a stroke that occurs as a result of a wandering clot or embolus that may become lodged in a cerebral artery and thus reduce or cut off the blood supply to the area of the brain beyond the clot. In practically all cerebral embolisms, the clot begins in the heart, aorta, or other proximal large vessels.

The cerebral deficit associated with the embolism usually occurs very rapidly. The damage is worst at the beginning and usually does not increase in severity. However, there may be quick improvement in some patients because the embolus may dissolve or break up.

A cerebral embolism occurs most often in patients who are awake. A mild headache is usually the first symptom, with the other neurological signs and symptoms associated with a CVA following by several hours.

CEREBRAL HEMORRHAGE

A cerebral *hemorrhage* occurs when an artery ruptures and fills the **cranium** with blood, resulting in an increase in the pressure within the cranium. This increase in pressure can cause a displacement of the brain and ultimately death. Cerebral **edema**, swelling of the neural tissue, always develops and adds to the high death rate from this type of CVA.

The two main sources of cerebral hemorrhage are a ruptured **aneurysm** and hypertensive vascular disease. The rupture in both these cases usually occurs as a result of an abrupt change in systolic blood pressure. The stress and anxiety associated with various dental procedures can cause this rise in systolic pressure.

Although cerebral hemorrhage is seen most often in older patients, it may also occur in young patients as a result of a ruptured aneurysm or malformed blood vessel.

Several causes of a CVA take place while the patient is asleep. A cerebral hemorrhage usually occurs when the patient is awake and active, so it is not uncommon for this type of CVA to occur in the dental office.

Signs and symptoms may occur very quickly and then increase in severity over the next short period. Victims of a hemorrhage often complain of an excruciating headache. The headache is localized at first, but as the bleeding spreads, the headache too spreads. The headache associated with a hemorrhage occurs because the blood has an irritating effect on the neural tissues.

Other signs and symptoms include nausea and vomiting, chills and sweating, and dizziness. Severe neurologic deficit such as **hemoplegia** or coma may occur. The severity of the symptoms is usually related to the amount of intracranial bleeding.

On the average, one third of these patients lose consciousness within a few minutes of onset. This indicates that a large hemorrhage has occurred, and usually there is a poor prognosis.

CEREBRAL INFARCTION

Cerebral infarction is a type of CVA that occurs as a result of some problem in the arterial blood supply from the heart to the brain. This problem usually occurs as a result of *atherosclerosis*. In these cases there is a thickening in an artery, which causes a decrease in the amount of oxygenated blood going to a particular area of the brain.

Since this type of stroke is slow in developing, noticeable neurologic deficits are also slow in developing. Unlike most classes of CVAs, headache, nausea, and vomiting are usually not present. Furthermore, the patient usually awakens in the morning with neurologic deficits from the **ischemia** that occurred during the night. *deficiency of blood supply*

CEREBRAL THROMBOSIS

The last main cause of CVA is a cerebral thrombosis, which occurs when there is an obstruction of the cerebral artery by a clot that forms within that artery. This differs from an embolism, in which the clot forms in another area of the body.

Atherosclerosis is a main cause of cerebral thrombosis. To prevent cerebral thrombosis, it is extremely important to treat aggressively conditions associated with atherosclerosis such as **hypertension**.

Like cerebral infarction, thrombosis very commonly happens during sleep and the patient awakens with the resulting signs of a stroke. Signs such as stuttering or other gradual deficits that reach their maximum in one to three days are often associated with thrombosis.

Although it is beneficial for the dental auxiliary to understand the various causes of a CVA, it is not necessary to distinguish between them to provide proper emergency treatment. Emergency treatment is basically the same for all causes of CVAs.

SIGNS AND SYMPTOMS

Signs and symptoms of a CVA vary, depending on the area affected and the type of CVA. Specific signs and symptoms of the various causes of a CVA were covered earlier. However, some similar signs and symptoms are usually seen when the dental patient experiences a CVA:

1. Headache may be the first symptom in several types, but other neurological signs and symptoms will soon develop.
2. Unconsciousness may occur. This is usually an ominous sign and indicates a severe stroke.
3. Paralysis may occur in the extremities of both sides, although it is most often unilateral.
4. Conscious patients may appear confused and have difficulty in understanding where they are or what has happened.

EMERGENCY BASICS

Signs and Symptoms of CVA

- Headache
- Unconsciousness
- Paralysis
- Confusion
- Impaired speech
- Unequal pupils
- Respiratory difficulty

5. Speech is usually impaired as a result of paralysis in some of the facial muscles or in the areas of the brain associated with speech.
6. The pupils of the eyes are usually of unequal size, a sign evident in both the conscious and unconscious patient.
7. The patient may experience difficulty in breathing.

TREATMENT

If a CVA occurs while the patient is in the dental office, the dental team should not waste time trying to determine the cause; the same emergency treatment is administered regardless.

If the dental team recognizes the signs and symptoms of a CVA, it should be most concerned with monitoring the patient's respiratory and circulatory status. It is important to make sure the airway is open and adequate oxygen is available, since the patient is already suffering from an oxygen deficiency.

Specifically, treatment should include:

1. Stop all dental treatment. Be sure to remove all objects from in and around the patient's mouth.
2. Position the patient with the head slightly elevated to relieve intracranial pressure.
3. Monitor the vital signs. This will provide helpful information for the paramedic unit.

EMERGENCY BASICS

Treatment of CVA

1. Stop all dental treatment
2. Position the patient
3. Monitor vital signs
4. Administer oxygen
5. Summon medical assistance
6. Keep the patient calm and quiet
7. Provide basic life support as needed
8. Do not administer drugs that alter neurological activity

4. Administer oxygen. The patient is suffering from an oxygen deficiency, so this helps to make the patient more comfortable.
5. Summon medical assistance. This patient requires more extensive treatment than the dental team is able to provide. It is of utmost importance that the patient be transported to a medical facility as soon as possible.
6. Keep the patient calm and quiet. It is important that the patient not become overheated or upset, since this can hasten brain damage.
7. Be prepared to provide basic life support. At any point is may become necessary to perform CPR, and the dental team should be prepared for this at all times.
8. No medication should be given that could affect the hospital's ability to determine the changes in neurological ability.

Any time the dental team deals with someone who has experienced a CVA, it must keep in mind that the person may die at any time; resuscitation efforts will not help because there has been extensive brain damage. Nevertheless, if it becomes necessary, the dental team must always attempt to resuscitate the patient.

Furthermore, even though CVA patients may not be able to speak, if they are conscious they are probably able to hear everything that is said, so the dental team must be very careful not to say anything that might upset the patient.

SUMMARY

Fortunately, a CVA is not a common occurrence in the dental office. It nevertheless can occur, and the dental team must be prepared to treat such patients. As with all emergencies, the best treatment is prevention. The dental team can best achieve this by realizing that certain people are prone to CVAs. For example, diabetics, those suffering from hypertension, those with a history of cardiac disease, and those with a history of TIAs are more likely to experience a CVA in the dental office than other patients are.

Furthermore, people who survive a CVA are at a high risk of recurrence. If the dental team is treating a post-CVA patient or a patient prone to experience a first-time CVA, extreme care must be taken to control anxiety and pain, which could easily trigger a CVA.

A CVA is a difficult emergency for the dental team to treat. It is best to do everything possible to prevent a CVA and be totally prepared to provide the best treatment possible should one occur.

REFERENCES

Ellison, Jeffrey P. "Cerebrovascular Disease: Evaluation and Management." *Consultant* (June 1981).

Edmeads, John. "Strategies in Stroke." *Emergency Medicine* (February 28, 1983).

Friedlander, A.H., Friedlander, I. K. "Identification of stroke prone patients by panoramic radiography." *Australian Dental Journal 43 (1)*, 51–54. February 1998.

Garcia-Monco, J.C., Capelastequi, A., Beldarrin, M. G., & Guerra, E. (1997) "Cerebrovascular accident in a 77 year-old man." *Postgraduate Medical Journal 73*, 251–253. April 1997.

Grant, Harvey, and Robert Murray. *Emergency Care*. Robert J. Brady Co., 1978.

Malamed, Stanley F. *Handbook of Medical Emergencies in the Dental Office*. 2nd ed. St. Louis: Mosby, 1982.

McCarthy, Frank M. *Medical Emergencies in Dentistry*. Philadelphia: Saunders, 1982.

Tyler, Kenneth L., and H. Richard Tyler. "Answers to Questions on Stroke: Part I." *Hospital Medicine* (July 1983).

Tyler, Kenneth L., and H. Richard Tyler. "Answers to Questions About Stroke: Part II." *Hospital Medicine* (August 1983).

REVIEW QUESTIONS

MULTIPLE CHOICE

1. A stroke that only exhibits signs and symptoms for a few minutes is known as a
   a. RIND
   b. cerebral embolism
   c. cerebral infarction
   d. none of the above

2. A stroke that occurs as a result of a clot forming in some area of the body and traveling to the brain is known as a:
   a. cerebral infarction
   b. cerebral embolism
   c. cerebral thrombosis
   d. TIA

3. What type of stroke is most likely to occur in the dental office?
   a. cerebral hemorrhage
   b. cerebral embolism
   c. cerebral infarction
   d. all the above

4. Which of the following conditions may result in a cerebral hemorrhage?
   1. aneurysm
   2. emboli
   3. hypertensive vascular disease
   4. ischemia
      a. 1, 2, 3
      b. 1, 3, 4
      c. 1, 2
      d. 1, 3

5. Cerebral thrombosis occurs most often as a result of:
   a. atherosclerosis
   b. aneurysm
   c. embolism
   d. none of the above

6. A patient suffering from a stroke should be positioned:
   a. in the Trendelenburg position
   b. in the supine position
   c. upright
   d. with the head slightly elevated

7. Which of the following patients have increased chances of experiencing a CVA?
   1. hypertensive
   2. diabetic
   3. history of heart disease
   4. history of TIA
      a. 1, 2, 3
      b. 2, 3
      c. 1, 4
      d. 1, 2, 3, 4

8. Which of the following are signs or symptoms of a CVA?
   1. headache
   2. paralysis
   3. nausea
   4. dizziness
      a. 1, 2
      b. 1, 2, 3
      c. 2, 4
      d. 1, 2, 3, 4

9. Which of the following is/are included in the emergency treatment of a CVA?
   1. administer a CNS relaxer
   2. maintain an open airway
   3. administer oxygen
   4. summon medical assistance
      a. 1, 2, 3, 4
      b. 1, 2, 4
      c. 2, 3, 4
      d. 1, 3, 4

10. Signs and symptoms associated with a cerebral hemorrhage include:
    1. vertigo
    2. vomiting
    3. stupor
    4. difficulty in movement
       a. 1, 3, 4
       b. 4
       c. 1, 2, 3, 4
       d. 2, 3

TRUE OR FALSE

F   1. TIAs usually last at least 48 hours.
T   2. Cerebral embolisms usually occur while the patient is awake.
T   3. A cerebral hemorrhage is usually preceded by a headache.
T   4. A cerebral thrombosis occurs as a result of an obstruction of the cerebral artery by a clot that forms within the artery.
F   5. It is imperative that the dental team know what caused the CVA before it can provide proper treatment.
T   6. Paralysis associated with a CVA is usually unilateral.
T   7. Signs and symptoms of a CVA vary according to the area of the brain affected as well as the type of CVA.
F   8. People who survive a CVA experience a low risk of recurrence.
T   9. Anxiety and pain associated with a dental appointment have the potential to trigger a CVA.
F 10. It is uncommon for a patient to experience a TIA prior to experiencing a severe stroke.

■ CASE STUDY

Mary Edmunds is 45 years old and in good general health. She documents on the health history that she has had repeated episodes of TIAs. While in the office she loses consciousness, then regains consciousness but is unable to speak. The dentist determines that the patient is experiencing a CVA.

QUESTIONS

1. State the signs and symptoms of a CVA.
2. State the treatment that will be performed for this patient.

Occupational Hazards and Emergencies

13

KEY TERMS

Endodontic file
Endodontic reamer

Herpes simplex virus
Ionizing radiation

OBJECTIVES

Upon completion of this chapter, the student will be able to:

- Define AIDS
- Explain ways the dental team can prevent the transmission of AIDS
- Define herpetic whitlow
- Explain how the dental team can avoid contracting herpetic whitlow
- Explain the hazards of mercury contamination
- Explain how to prevent mercury contamination
- Explain how to avoid the transmission of hepatitis B
- Describe how to avoid the hazards of ionizing radiation
- Describe how to prevent breakage of an anesthetic needle

- Explain the treatment needed to remove a broken endodontic file or reamer
- Explain how the auxiliary can help prevent soft-tissue injuries
- Define alveolitis
- Explain the treatment for alveolitis
- Describe ways to prevent the patient from aspirating foreign objects
- Describe the hazards of nitrous oxide oxygen sedation

Most emergencies in the dental office occur as a result of some associated medical condition. However, some emergencies occur as a result of the dental treatment itself, and there are conditions in the dental office that present hazards to the dental personnel as well.

The first section of this chapter covers potential hazards present in the office that have the potential to injure the office personnel. The second section presents a few of the more common emergencies that may arise as a result of certain dental procedures.

HAZARDS TO OFFICE PERSONNEL

Acquired Immune Deficiency Syndrome

Since the discovery of acquired immune deficiency syndrome (AIDS) in the late 1970s, more and more cases have been reported. With the increase in cases the potential for the dental team to come in contact with either a diag-

EMERGENCY BASICS

Increased Risk Group for AIDS

Homosexual or bisexual men
Drug abusers using IV injections
Hemophiliacs
Sexual partners of AIDS victims
Children of these high-risk populations

nosed or undiagnosed AIDS victim also increases. It is therefore important for the auxiliary to be aware of this disease and the possible cross-contamination that could affect the dental team.

AIDS is characterized by a distinct defect in cell-mediated immunity that leaves the victim vulnerable to an unlimited number of infections and neoplasms. People suffering from AIDS usually experience a great deal of pain and suffering as well as an extremely high mortality rate.

The transmission routes of AIDS are of concern to the dental auxiliary. Based on epidemiological evidence, it is likely that AIDS is transmitted either by intimate sexual contact or parenteral inoculation. In order to protect the dental team from any risk, the guidelines stated in the OSHA Bloodborne Pathogen Standard should always be followed. There is still a great deal that is unknown about AIDS. And since with increasing cases the dental office may encounter an AIDS victim, it is important for the auxiliary to recognize AIDS as a potential hazard and treat it accordingly.

Herpetic Whitlow

Prior to treating a patient, the dental auxiliary notices a small sore above the patient's lip. What the auxiliary may not realize is that he is about to be exposed to the **herpes simplex virus**. Herpes simplex virus has the potential to be spread from the infected patient to the dental team and thus infect such areas as the eyes or mouth. However, as far as dental personnel are concerned, the most common infected area is the hand or finger. This condition is termed herpetic whitlow and is a known occupational hazard.

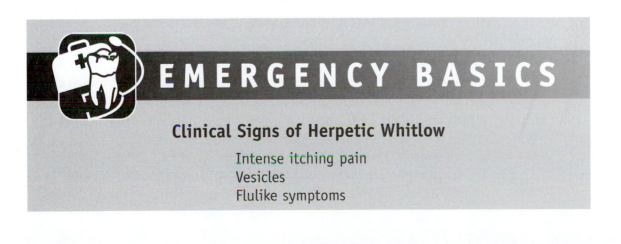

EMERGENCY BASICS

Clinical Signs of Herpetic Whitlow

Intense itching pain
Vesicles
Flulike symptoms

Clinical features of herpetic whitlow include intense itching pain and vesicles with fluid that may be clear at first but later appears yellow; flulike symptoms may also be present.

To eliminate the possibility of contracting the herpes simplex virus, the auxiliary should implement the following steps:

1. Wear a mask, gloves, and safety glasses.
2. In some situations the dentist may prefer to reappoint the patient after the virus is no longer active. However, this decision should always be made by the dentist, not the auxiliary.
3. Utilize a dental dam. This eliminates direct contact between the lesion and the dental team's hands.
4. All instruments should then be sterilized, disposable items removed, and surface area disinfected.

Mercury Contamination

Practically all dental offices deal with mercury on a daily basis. Because of the potentially toxic effects of mercury poisoning, mercury hygiene should be an important consideration for the dental team.

Mercury can be absorbed through the skin if the auxiliary handles it improperly during the preparation of amalgam. However, mercury is absorbed mainly by inhalation of vapors in the air. Mercury vapors can be released into the air by improperly storing scrap amalgam, by spilling mercury in the operatory, and by removing old amalgam with a high-speed handpiece without water.

Mercury poisoning can cause birth defects, brain dysfunction, kidney problems, and other associated conditions. In addition, mercury poisoning is extremely dangerous because the dental team may never be aware that an office is contaminated until serious effects have taken place.

To prevent mercury poisoning the following precautions should be taken:

1. Never touch the amalgam or mercury with bare hands.
2. Enclose scrap amalgam in a tight container with used x-ray fixer or a specially prepared mercury solution that can be purchased from most supply companies. (At one time it was suggested that scrap amalgam be stored in water, but we now know that water does not prevent the emission of mercury vapors.)
3. Try to prevent all mercury spills. If a spill does occur, special techniques should be followed. Always use one of the several devices that

can be purchased for the purpose to collect a spill. Never collect a mercury spill with the high-speed suction or a vacuum cleaner.

4. When removing an old amalgam, always use water with the high-speed handpiece. The suction should always be placed close to the operative site to catch any debris or dust removed from the tooth.

5. Most state governmental agencies have departments that will come into the dental office to monitor mercury levels upon request. This should be done on a routine basis.

Mercury, then, has potential for causing serious problems within the dental office. However, if handled properly, mercury need not be an occupational hazard.

Hepatitis B

Hepatitis B is probably the best-known occupational hazard for dental personnel. As a matter of fact, it has been recognized as such a major problem that a hepatitis vaccine has been developed.

Hepatitis B affects the liver. The disease itself is a real problem, but for the dental team a special problem is that a person may remain a carrier of the disease for an indefinite period. Dentists or auxiliaries may not be able to practice dentistry for a prolonged period if they are diagnosed as being carriers of hepatitis B. Hepatitis B can be transmitted by infected blood, saliva, and other body fluids. It is a distinct occupational hazard for dental personnel, since they constantly deal with saliva and blood.

To prevent this potential hazard from becoming a true health problem, the dental team must prevent the transmission of the virus from the infected patient to the dental team. This is accomplished by implementing the following steps:

1. Take the hepatitis B vaccine.
2. Maintain a thorough, updated medical history on each patient.
3. Wear a mask, gloves, and safety glasses.
4. Wrap areas such as light handles with aluminum foil. It can be thrown away after the appointment, and these hard-to-clean areas will not be contaminated.
5. Use disposable items whenever possible.
6. Take special care when cleaning and preparing instruments for sterilization. Any auxiliary cut by one of the contaminated instruments should notify a physician for immediate treatment.
7. Sterilize all instruments.

8. Clean counters and cabinet tops with a solution known to kill the hepatitis virus.

A special problem associated with hepatitis B is that a person may become a carrier without ever actually having the disease and transmit it without even being aware of doing so. To adequately protect themselves and their patients, the dental team should implement the steps above for all patients.

Radiation

Dental radiation, used properly, is one of the most beneficial of diagnostic tools available, but used carelessly it is a potential occupational hazard.

The damaging effects of **ionizing radiation** are widely known. Some auxiliaries, however, are not aware of the situations that place them in danger when they are exposed to excessive amounts of radiation. To prevent this exposure, the auxiliary should:

1. Never stay in the room when a radiograph is being exposed unless there is a lead-lined screen to stand behind while exposing the radiograph.
2. Always be at least six feet away from the x-ray head, which will place the technician out of the range of the x-ray beam.
3. Never hold the film in the patient's mouth.
4. Wear a personal monitoring device. This usually takes the form of a badge that monitors the amounts of radiation to which an auxiliary is exposed. These may be purchased through several different companies. The badges are returned each month to the company, which monitors and reports the amount of radiation exposure, if any.

Radiation, as well as the other topics in this section, have the potential to become occupational hazards. However, when treated carefully, most hazards can be eliminated or rendered harmless.

PATIENT DENTAL EMERGENCIES

This section describes some of the emergency situations that may occur in the office as a result of dental treatment. Many dentistry-related emergencies can occur, but this section is limited to those that seem to occur most often.

Broken Anesthetic Needle

An anesthetic needle may be broken during an injection because of poor technique by the dentist, a needle imperfection, or an abrupt violent movement by the patient. This kind of emergency occurs more often during a mandibular injection because of the position of the needle.

If this emergency should occur, the patient should be informed of the situation by the dentist. The auxiliary should do everything possible to help keep the patient calm. Removal of a broken needle can be a complicated surgical procedure. Therefore, unless the dentist has extensive surgical experience, he or she usually refers the patient to an oral surgeon.

The auxiliary can help prevent this emergency by examining the needle before the injection and by keeping the patient from grabbing or hitting the dentist's hand during the injection.

If this emergency should occur, the auxiliary should record the entire incident in the patient's chart. This may prove valuable should later legal action be taken.

Separated Endodontic Reamer or File

During root canal therapy, a root canal or **endodontic file** or **reamer** may separate and remain the periapical area. To prevent further complications the dentist must remove this fragment. The auxiliary must be prepared to assist with any procedure the dentist chooses.

Soft-tissue Injury

During surgical procedures it is very common for the surgical site to become very slippery and consequently easy for a sharp surgical instrument to slip off the tooth and lacerate the surrounding soft tissues.

This may wound the tongue, cheek, or gingival areas. The dentist treats each area as required, and the auxiliary should be prepared to assist with any necessary procedure.

In some situations the auxiliary can help prevent laceration of the soft tissue by proficient suctioning, which keeps the area clear and increases visibility. The auxiliary may also use a mirror or other instrument to retract the tongue from the surgical area.

Alveolitis

Alveolitis, also known as dry socket, is a very common and uncomfortable post-surgical complication that occurs when a blood clot does not form or is washed out of a surgical socket. Since there is no clot, the nerve endings in the bone are exposed, which results in extreme pain and also opens the area to risk of infection.

The main goal of treatment in this case is to make the patient comfortable. The auxiliary can assist the dentist within the limits of state regulations and may help prevent alveolitis by instructing the patient in correct postoperative care.

Aspiration of a Foreign Object

The dental office is the perfect setting for the aspiration of an object into the airway. The patient is supine, the saliva makes everything slippery, and the dental team is constantly placing small objects in and removing them from the patient's mouth.

A few common objects aspirated by patients include crowns, bridges, dental-dam clamps, and burs. The auxiliary can play an important role in preventing the aspiration of each of these objects.

When trying in crowns, permanent or temporary, the auxiliary should unfold a 2 x 2 gauze and place it across the back of the throat, in front of the gag-reflex area, as a screen. If the crown is dropped, it will be caught in the gauze and can be easily removed. This same 2 x 2 gauze should be in place when extracting teeth to catch any pieces that may break.

If the dentist is trying in a bridge, the auxiliary should tie a 10- to 12-inch piece of floss around the pontic. The auxiliary can then hold onto the end of the floss while the dentist tries in the bridge.

When placing a dental-dam clamp, the auxiliary should tie a piece of floss around the clamp. The floss should then be held while the clamp is placed on the tooth. If the clamp slips off the tooth, the auxiliary will be holding the floss and it will not be aspirated (see Figure 13-1).

A dental bur can break at any time and a small part could be aspirated. This may be prevented by utilizing a rubber dam whenever possible. Furthermore, the auxiliary should always tug on the bur before it is used to make sure it is firmly placed in the handpiece.

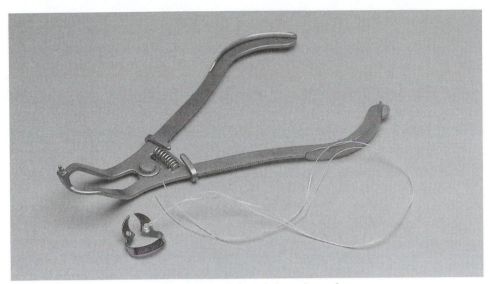

Figure 13-1 Clamp with floss safety ligature and dental dam clamp forceps.

Nitrous Oxide Oxygen Sedation

Nitrous sedation is being used more and more frequently in today's dental office. When used properly, it provides a more pleasant experience for most anxious dental patients. On the other hand, nitrous oxide can become a hazard not only to the patient but also to the dental team if it is used incorrectly.

Over the past few years it has become known that continuous exposure to nitrous vapors can be hazardous to dental personnel. When nitrous oxide is administered through a nosepiece, some amount of the gas leaks around the mask. In the past, the dental team was constantly inhaling these escaping vapors. Physical problems such as miscarriages and infertility have been noted to occur as a result of this exposure. Today's units have an attachment (known as a scavenger unit) that collects any excess gas. All units should have this attachment.

When administered at the proper dose and rate, nitrous oxide provides a very good sedative for the dental patient. However, if the dosage is incorrect, the substance becomes a general anesthetic and the patient loses consciousness, presenting a serious condition in the dental office that should always be avoided.

To achieve optimal effects from nitrous oxide, the dental team must properly explain its effects to the patient. The patient should know that he can reduce the effects of nitrous oxide by breathing through the mouth rather than through the nosepiece. The gas should then be introduced slowly. The dental team should keep constant conversation going during the beginning stages. Uncommunicative patients can suddenly become excited and have been known to injure themselves or dental personnel by suddenly jumping out of the chair. Too, the patient receiving nitrous oxide may vomit. This can create a potential problem is the patient aspirates the vomitus.

Nitrous oxide and oxygen sedation, when administered and monitored properly, can be used safely and effectively. However, the auxiliary should be aware that there are potential complications associated with the use of nitrous oxide.

SUMMARY

The dental office can present both the dental team and the patient with hazardous situations. The auxiliary should realize that most of these situations may be prevented if treated correctly. However, no matter what prevention techniques are employed, some emergencies will occur. It is these situations the auxiliary needs to know how to handle properly.

REFERENCES

Auci, Anthony S., and H. Clifford Lane. "Overview of Clinical Syndromes and Immunology of AIDS." *Topics in Clinical Nursing* (July 1984).

Cooley, Robert L., and Richard M. Bubow. "Hepatitis B Vaccine: Implications for Dental Personnel." *Journal of the American Dental Association 105* (July 1982).

Cooley, Robert L., and Wayne W. Barkmeier. "Techniques and Devices for Recovering Mercury and Preventing Contamination." *General Dentistry* (January-February 1982).

Henderson, David K. "AIDS: Epidemiology and Potential for Nosocomial Transmission." *Topics in Clinical Nursing* (July 1984).

Krammer, Howard S. Jr., and Von A Mitton. "Complications of Local Anesthesia." *Dental Clinics of North America 17* (July 1973).

LaCamera, Deborah. "AIDS: Precautions for Health Care Personnel." *Topics in Clinical Nursing* (July 1984).

Osbon, Donald B. "Postoperative Complications Following Dentoalveolar Surgery." *Dental Clinics of North America 17* (July 1973).

Rothstein, Sandford S., Harriet S. Goldman, and Anthony S. Arcomano. "Hepatitis B Virus: An Overview for Dentists." *Journal of the American Dental Association 102* (February 1981).

Rowe, Nathaniel H., Carol S. Heine, and Charles J. Kowalski. "Herpetic Whitlow: An Occupational Disease of Practicing Dentists." *Journal of the American Dental Association 105* (September 1982).

Trieger, Norman. "Emergencies and Complications from Sedation Modalities." *Dental Clinics of North America 17* (July 1973).

Vandenberge, John, Alan S. Moodie, and Ralph E. Keller, Jr. "Blood Serum Mercury Test Report." *Journal of the American Dental Association 94* (June 1977).

REVIEW QUESTIONS

MULTIPLE CHOICE

1. Which of the following people would be considered in the high-risk category for AIDS?
   a. hemophiliacs
   b. homosexual men
   c. sexual partners of AIDS victims
   d. all the above

2. Herpetic whitlow is a type of the herpes simplex virus that appears on the:
   a. finger
   b. lip
   c. eye
   d. tongue

3. Which of the following is not true concerning the handling of mercury?
   a. Mercury should never be touched with the hands.
   b. Scrap amalgam or mercury should be stored in a dry container.
   c. Water spray should be used when removing an old amalgam.
   d. Excess mercury should never be suctioned with the high-volume suction.

4. A condition that occurs when a clot does not form in an extraction site is:
   a. periodontitis
   b. cellulitis
   c. edema
   d. alveolitis

5. A disease characterized by a defect in cell-mediated immunity is known as:
   a. AIDS
   b. hepatitis B
   c. hepatitis A
   d. alveolitis

6. Which of the following is/are commonly associated with herpetic whitlow?
   a. flulike symptoms
   b. intense itching pain
   c. vesicles
   d. all the above

7. If the auxiliary must be in the room when the x-ray is being exposed, she should be:
   a. at the patient's feet
   b. behind a lead screen
   c. holding the tube head
   d. all the above

8. The auxiliary may prevent the breaking of an anesthetic needle by:
   a. using a larger-gauge needle
   b. keeping the patient from hitting the dentist's hands
   c. using a shorter needle
   d. all the above

9. For optimum protection from infectious diseases, the auxiliary should:
   a. wear a mask
   b. wear gloves
   c. wear safety glasses
   d. all the above

10. To eliminate constant exposure to nitrous oxide vapors, the dental team should use a unit that has a:
    a. scavenger unit
    b. full-mouth mask
    c. clear nosepiece
    d. none of the above

TRUE OR FALSE

F 1. AIDS is easily contracted by health care workers who are not in the high-risk group.

T 2. Hepatitis B may be transmitted by saliva.

T 3. A person may be a carrier of hepatitis B without ever having the disease.

F 4. A broken anesthetic needle occurs most often during maxillary injections.

F 5. A broken endodontic file does not need to be removed from the canal.

T 6. A 2 x 2 gauze should be placed at the back of the throat to prevent a crown from going down the throat during cementation.

F 7. A scavenger unit is not needed on today's nitrous oxide units.

T 8. A patient can reduce the effects of nitrous oxide by breathing through the mouth.

F 9. The prognosis for AIDS victims is very good.

T 10. Wearing mask, gloves, and safety glasses is important in preventing the transmission of all diseases.

■ CASE STUDY

Sheila Black is a 35-year-old patient. She has come to the dental office to have a crown placed on tooth number 3. The crown has been delivered from the lab and the dentist is preparing to try the crown on the tooth.

QUESTIONS

Describe what steps should be taken to prevent a possible airway obstruction from occurring during the try-in of the crown.

14

Legal Problems of Emergency Care

KEY TERMS

Abandonment
Negligence

OBJECTIVES

Upon completion of this chapter, the student will be able to:

- Explain the dental team's general legal duties to the patient
- Explain ways the dental team can prevent lawsuits against the dental team

This chapter is designed to provide the auxiliary with very basic information concerning legal problems associated with emergency care. Laws vary from state to state, and each auxiliary should check the laws pertaining to her own state. Furthermore, laws that could affect the outcome of a particular legal action are changing every day.

The number of lawsuits against health professionals is growing. To reduce such cases, the dental team must first understand its legal obligations to the patient.

DUTY TO TREAT

The dental team has an obligation, once it begins treatment, to provide all the treatment required by the patient. In an emergency, the dental team must do everything in its power to provide care for the patient. This treatment requirement also includes the transfer of the patient to a hospital if the scope of the emergency requires more extensive care than is available in the dental office.

DUTY NOT TO ABANDON

Once the dental team begins to treat the patient, it has a duty not to abandon the patient. In an emergency situation, this means the dentist must first stabilize the patient and then transfer the patient to a medical facility if necessary. If the dental team did not begin treatment on the patient but merely summoned transportation to a medical facility, the patient may have grounds for legal action. Furthermore, the dental team must never allow the patient to leave the dental office until the emergency is over. For example, if a patient complained of chest pains, was allowed by the dental team to leave while still experiencing the pain, and suffered from myocardial infarction, it is extremely possible that she could sue the dental team for negligence on the grounds of abandonment.

DUTY OF PREPAREDNESS

The dental team has a legal duty to the patient to be prepared for an emergency. First, the dental team must have the knowledge to administer basic care in the event of an emergency. Second, the office must contain basic emergency equipment such as an oxygen tank and a complete emergency kit. Third, the dentist must have a staff trained in basic emergency treatment.

A failure of the dental team to meet any of its legal duties leaves the team liable for lawsuits based mainly on negligence.

DENTAL STAFF'S RESPONSIBILITIES

The dentist is ultimately responsible for the actions of employees while they are at work. However, dental auxiliaries can still be held liable for their actions and included in any lawsuit against the dentist. Auxiliaries therefore have the legal obligation to be prepared for an emergency by being trained in emergency treatment such as CPR.

GOOD SAMARITAN LAW

Most states have enacted Good Samaritan Laws. These laws give legal protection to people who provide emergency care to ill or injured people.

Good Samaritan Laws were developed to encourage people to help others in emergency situations. They require that the "Good Samaritan" use common sense and a reasonable level of skill, not to exceed the scope of the individual's training in emergency situations. They assume each person would do his or her best to save a life or prevent further injury.

People are rarely sued for helping in emergency. However, the existence of Good Samaritan Laws does not mean that someone cannot sue. In rare court cases, courts have ruled that these laws do not apply in cases when an individual rescuer's action was grossly or willfully negligent or reckless or when the rescuer abandoned the victim after initiating care.

Dental office staff should always be current in their CPR and emergency training and be prepared to assist a patient in the event of an emergency.

PREVENTING LEGAL PROBLEMS

The dental team cannot prevent every emergency. Similarly, the dental team cannot prevent a patient from bringing legal actions. However, the dental team can do several things to prevent the patient from being successful if there is litigation.

First, the dental team must do everything possible to prevent an emergency from occurring. This can be achieved by utilizing optimum, updated dental techniques; by maintaining updated medical histories; and by having the necessary knowledge and equipment to handle an emergency.

Second, the dental team should establish an emergency routine and practice it on a regular basis.

Third, the dental office should have all emergency numbers available near the phone. One office member should be designated to summon medical assistance when needed.

Finally, should an emergency occur, the auxiliary should write, in detail, everything that transpired prior to, during, and after the emergency. This will prove extremely important if a patient sues, enabling the defense to present the court with the pertinent facts of the emergency.

SUMMARY

Patients can initiate lawsuits against any member of the dental team. Each state's legal requirements for the dental team differ. It is important for the dental team to be aware of its responsibilities. By being aware of those responsibilities, the dental team will be better prepared to prevent legal actions or to answer them.

REFERENCES

Holzapfel, George S. "Legal Aspects of Emergency Dental Care." *Dental Clinics of North America 26* (January 1982).

McCarthy, Frank M. *Medical Emergencies in Dentistry.* Philadelphia: Saunders. 1982.

Ursu, Samuel C. "The Medical Malpractice Dilemma." *Dental Clinics of North America 26* (April 1982).

Zinman, Edward J. "Legal Aspects of Medical Emergencies in the Dental Office." *Dental Management* (May 1983).

■ CASE STUDY

Molly Blazer is a 45-year-old female. She has come to the dental office for a check-up and cleaning. During the appointment, Ms. Blazer experiences chest pains. The dental team determines that Ms. Blazer is possibly experiencing a heart attack. They provide treatment for the patient and call for emergency medical assistance. Ms. Blazer is transported to the hospital.

QUESTION

What should the dental team complete once the patient is stabilized and transported to the hospital? Why?

■ Glossary

ABANDONMENT
Wrongful cessation of the provision of care to a patient.

ABDOMINAL THRUSTS
Technique used as part of the Heimlich maneuver which uses abdominal thrusts to try to dislodge an object.

ALLERGEN
Any substance capable of inducing an allergic reaction.

AMPULE
Sealed glass container that holds a single dose of medication.

AMYL NITRITE
A vasodilator.

ANAPHYLAXIS
A severe life-threatening allergic reaction.

ANEURYSM
Abnormality of a blood vessel, usually an artery, caused most often by a defect or weakness of the wall of the vessel.

ANGINA PECTORIS
A severe pain in and around the heart caused by an insufficient supply of oxygenated blood to the heart.

ANGIOEDEMA
An allergic reaction characterized by swelling of the skin or mucous membrane.

ANTIBODY
A protein produced to react specifically with an antigen.

ANTICOAGULANT
Agent used to prevent coagulation of the blood.

ANTICUBITAL FOSSA
Area approximately one inch from the elbow in which the stethoscope is placed in order to hear the pulse when measuring blood pressure.

ANTIGEN
Substance that causes the formation of an antibody.

ANTIHISTAMINE
A drug used to combat the reactions of histamine.

AORTA
Main artery of the human body.

ARTERIOSCLEROSIS
Thickening of the artery walls that results in loss of elasticity.

ARTIFICIAL RESPIRATION
The process of artificially maintaining respiration when normal breathing has stopped.

ASPHYXIATION
Death caused by lack of oxygen.

ASPIRATE
To breathe in forcefully causing an object to become lodged in the airway.

ASTHMA
An affliction of the respiratory tract that can affect all aspects of the tracheobronchial tree.

ATHEROSCLEROSIS
Form of arteriosclerosis that affects the coronary arteries and causes coronary artery disease.

ATRIA
Upper chambers of the heart.

ATRIOVENTRICULAR VALVE
A valve in the heart through which blood flows from the atria to the ventricles.

AURA
A sight, sound, or smell unique to an individual before experiencing an epileptic seizure.

BLOOD PRESSURE
The pressure the blood exerts on the walls of the arteries, the veins, and the chambers of the heart.

BRACHIAL ARTERY
The principal artery of the upper arm.

BRONCHITIS
An inflammation of the bronchi.

BRONCHODILATOR
A medication that dilates the bronchioles.

CARBON DIOXIDE
A colorless, odorless gas produced by the oxidation of carbon.

CARDIAC ARREST
When the heart has stopped.

CARDIAC ARRHYTHMIAS
Abnormal rhythms of the heart.

CAROTID ARTERY
Artery located on either side of the neck; used to measure the pulse during an emergency.

CEREBROVASCULAR ACCIDENT (CVA; commonly called a stroke)
A specific neurologic deficit that occurs suddenly as a result of vascular disease of a hemorrhagic or ischemic nature.

CLONIC
Movements associated with a grand mal seizure.

CONTACT DERMATITIS
Inflammation of the skin from contact with a sensitizing agent.

CRANIUM
The part of the skull that houses the brain.

CRICOTHYROTOMY
Incision made through the cricoid cartilage to relive an airway obstruction.

CYANOSIS
Bluish skin color that results from decreased oxygen.

DEMAND-VALVE RESUSCITATOR
Attachment for the oxygen tank that can force oxygen into the lungs of a nonbreathing victim.

DENTAL-DAM
A thin sheet of latex rubber for isolating one or more teeth during a dental procedure.

DIABETIC COMA
A life-threatening condition caused by a lack of insulin in the body.

DIABETIC RETINOPATHY
A disease of the retina that is a result of diabetes.

DIASTOLIC PRESSURE
Pressure on the arteries when the heart relaxes between beats.

DIAZEPAM
A medication used for the treatment of epilepsy.

DILANTIN
An anticonvulsant drug.

DILANTIN HYPERPLASIA
Overgrowth of gingival tissue that results from the intake of dilantin.

EDEMA
Local or generalized swelling from retention of excessive fluid.

EMBOLISM
A clot that forms somewhere in the body and travels throughout the body until it lodges.

EMBOLUS
A mass in the blood that was brought there by the blood or lymph.

EMERGENCY KIT
A kit containing the necessary medications and equipment required to treat an emergency.

ENDOCARDIUM
Lining of the inner heart surface.

ENDODONTIC FILE
A dental instrument used to remove the contents of the pulp chamber.

ENDODONTIC REAMER
A dental instrument used to remove the contents of the pulp chamber.

EPICARDIUM
Inner layer of the pericardium.

EPIGASTRIUM
Area of the upper abdomen.

EPIGLOTTIS
Structure that prevents food from entering the larynx and directs it into the esophagus.

EPINEPHRINE
A vasoconstrictor.

ERYTHEMA
Redness of the skin.

ESOPHAGUS
Tube that carries food from the pharynx to the stomach.

EXTERNAL COMPRESSION
Outside pressure placed on the lower sternum in order to force the blood out of the heart.

EXTRINSIC ASTHMA
A form of asthma caused by the exposure of the bronchial mucosa to an inhaled airborne antigen.

FLOWMETER
Attachment on the oxygen tank that controls the amount of oxygen that is delivered to the patient.

GANGRENE
Necrosis of tissue due to deficient or nonexistent blood supply.

GASTRIC DISTENTION
Enlargement of the stomach due to an increase of air being forced into it. Usually seen as a result of forceful artificial respiration.

GESTATIONAL DIABETES
Diabetes that usually occurs first during pregnancy.

GLUCAGON
A hormone produced in the pancreas that raises blood sugar.

GLUCOSE
Fuel for the body manufactured from the food one eats.

GOOD SAMARITAN LAW
A law which was designed to provide protection against prosecution for individuals that attempt to provide aid to someone during an emergency.

GRAND MAL SEIZURE
An epileptic seizure characterized by a generalized involuntary muscular contraction and cessation of respiration followed by tonic and clonic spasms of the muscles.

HEIMLICH MANEUVER
Technique used to remove an object that is lodged in the airway.

HEMIPLEGIA
Paralysis of one side of the body.

HEMOPHILIA
Hereditary blood disease characterized by prolonged coagulation time.

HEMORRHAGE
A great amount of loss of blood in a short period of time.

HERPES SIMPLEX VIRUS
A virus which has an affinity for the skin and nervous system.

HISTAMINE
Substance normally found in the body; its functions include increasing gastric secretions, constriction of the smooth muscles of the bronchioles, and dilation of capillaries.

HYPERGLYCEMIA
A condition that occurs when there is too much glucose in the blood.

HYPERTENSION (commonly known as high blood pressure)
Abnormally high pressure of the blood against the arterial walls.

HYPERVENTILATION
A respiratory emergency commonly seen in the dental office characterized by rapid breathing that results in a decrease in carbon dioxide.

HYPOGLYCEMIA (also called insulin shock)
A condition that occurs as a result of too little glucose in the body.

HYPOXIA
Oxygen deficiency.

IMMUNE SYSTEM
A biological complex that protects the body against pathogenic organisms and other foreign bodies.

IMMUNOGLOBULIN SYSTEM
Five structurally and antigenically distinct antibodies present in the serum and external secretions of the body.

INSULIN
Hormone secreted by the pancreas.

INSULIN SHOCK
A life-threatening condition caused by an excess of insulin in the body.

INTRINSIC ASTHMA
A nonallergic form of asthma usually first occurring later in life that tends to be chronic and persistent rather than episodic.

IONIZING RADIATION
High energy electromagnetic waves such as x-rays.

ISCHEMIA
Deficiency of blood supply.

KETONES
Normal metabolic products from which acetone may arise spontaneously.

LARYNGEAL EDEMA
Swelling of the larynx, often the result of an allergic reaction.

LARYNGECTOMY
Excision of the larynx.

MACROVASCULAR DISEASE
Disease of the large vessels.

MANDIBLE
Lower jaw.

MICROVASCULAR DISEASE
Disease of the small vessels of the body.

MYOCARDIAL INFARCTION
Circulatory emergency caused by occlusion of at least one of the coronary arteries.

MYOCARDIUM
Middle layer of the heart wall.

NASAL CANULA
An attachment that can be used with the oxygen tank which fits into the patient's nostrils and delivers the oxygen.

NEGLIGENCE
The omission of duty that results in injury or harm to another person.

NEOPLASM
Growth or tumor.

NEURONS
Conducting cells of the nervous system.

NITROGLYCERIN
A coronary vasodilator frequently prescribed for the prevention or relief of angina.

NONPSYCHOGENIC
Physical, nonpsychological causes of a condition.

ORAL HYPOGLYCEMICS
Medication that can lower blood sugar.

ORTHOSTATIC HYPOTENSION
Decrease in blood pressure when a person is raised supine to erect.

OXYGEN TANK
A cylinder that contains the oxygen.

PANCREAS
Body organ that produces insulin.

PARTIAL SEIZURE
Convulsive movements associated with epilepsy occur on one side of the body only.

PERICARDIUM
Sac that encloses the heart.

PERIODONTAL DISEASE
Disease of the periodontium.

PETIT MAL SEIZURE
An epileptic seizure characterized by a sudden momentary loss of consciousness occasionally accompanied by minor twitching.

PHARYNX
Passageway by which air travels from the nose to the larynx and food from the mouth to the esophagus.

PHYSICIAN'S DESK REFERENCE
Published document that provides information on various drugs.

PRESYNCOPE
First stage of syncope; stage prior to the actual loss of consciousness.

PSYCHOGENIC
Psychological causes of a condition.

PULMONARY ARTERY
Artery that runs from the right ventricle to the lungs.

PULSE
The regular expansion and contraction of an artery caused by the ejection of the blood from the left ventricle of the heart as it contracts.

RADIAL ARTERY
An artery located in the forearm.

REGULATOR
Attachment on an oxygen tank that allows oxygen to be released from the tank to the face mask or nasal canula.

REGURGITATION
Vomiting.

RESPIRATION RATE
The number of times that a person inhales and exhales.

SEMILUNAR VALVE
A valve with half moon shaped cusps like the aortic valve and the pulmonary valve.

SPHYGMOMANOMETER
Instrument that consists of a gauge and an inflatable bag inside an armband; used to measure blood pressure.

STATUS ASTHMATICUS
A severe form of asthma in which the victim experiences a continuous asthma attack.

STATUS EPILEPTICUS
Situation in which the victim experiences one seizure after another or one continuous seizure.

STERNUM
Narrow, flat bone located at the midline of the thorax.

STETHOSCOPE
Instrument used to listen to the heart and chest sounds.

STOMA
A small opening.

SUPINE POSITION
Lying horizontally on the back.

SYNCOPE
Fainting.

SYSTOLIC PRESSURE
Pressure on the arteries when the heart is beating, or working.

THROMBOSIS
A clot that forms in a vessel.

TRACHEA (also called the windpipe)
The air passage that descends from the larynx and branches into the right and left bronchi.

TRACHEOBRONCHIAL TREE
The trachea, bronchi, and the bronchial tubes.

TRACHEOTOMY
Incision made through the skin into the trachea to relieve an airway obstruction.

TRENDELENBURG POSITION
Position in which the patient is a supine with the feet higher than the head.

URTICARIA
A skin reaction characterized by the eruption of itching wheals.

VASODEPRESSOR SYNCOPE (also known as the common faint)
Loss of consciousness caused by a decrease in the blood flow to the brain.

VASODILATOR
An agent that causes the dilation of blood vessels.

VENTRICLES
Lower chambers of the heart.

VENTRICULAR FIBRILLATION
Spasmodic movement of the heart.

XIPHOID PROCESS
Lowest portion of the sternum.

■ Index